Equine Medical Disorders

LIBRARY OF VETERINARY PRACTICE

EDITORS

C. J. PRICE MA, VetMB, MRCVS
Hampden Veterinary Hospital
49 Cambridge Street
Aylesbury, Bucks

P. G. C. BEDFORD BVetMed, PhD, DVOphthal, FRCVS
Royal Veterinary College
Hawkshead Lane, North Mymms, Hatfield, Herts

J. B. SUTTON JP, MRCVS
2 Friarswood Road
Newcastle-under-Lyme, Staffs

LIBRARY OF VETERINARY PRACTICE

Equine Medical Disorders

A. M. JOHNSTON

BVM&S, DVetMed, MRCVS, FRSH

Senior Lecturer
Royal Veterinary College
Hatfield, Hertfordshire

SECOND EDITION

OXFORD

BLACKWELL SCIENTIFIC PUBLICATIONS

LONDON EDINBURGH BOSTON

MELBOURNE PARIS BERLIN VIENNA

© 1986, 1994 by
Blackwell Scientific Publications
Editorial Offices:
Osney Mead, Oxford OX2 0EL
25 John Street, London WC1N 2BL
23 Ainslie Place, Edinburgh EH3 6AJ
238 Main Street, Cambridge,
  Massachusetts, 02142, USA
54 University Street, Carlton,
  Victoria 3053, Australia

Other Editorial Offices:
Librairie Arnette SA
1, rue de Lille
75007 Paris
France

Blackwell Wissenschafts-Verlag GmbH
Düsseldorfer Str. 38
D-10707 Berlin
Germany

Blackwell MZV
Feldgasse 13
A-1238 Wien
Austria

First edition published 1986
Reprinted 1989
Second edition published 1994

Set by DP Photosetting, Aylesbury, Bucks
Printed and bound in Great Britain by
Hartnolls Ltd, Bodmin, Cornwall

DISTRIBUTORS

  Marston Book Services Ltd
  PO Box 87
  Oxford OX2 0DT
  (*Orders:* Tel: 0865 791155
          Fax: 0865 791927
          Telex: 837515)

USA
  Blackwell Scientific Publications, Inc.
  238 Main Street
  Cambridge, MA 02142
  (*Orders:* Tel: 800 759-6102
             617 876-7000)

Canada
  Times Mirror Professional Publishing, Ltd
  130 Flaska Drive
  Markham
  Ontario L6G 1B8
  (*Orders:* Tel: 800 268-4178
             416 470-6739)

Australia
  Blackwell Scientific Publications Pty Ltd
  54 University Street
  Carlton, Victoria 3053
  (*Orders:* Tel: 03 347-5552)

A catalogue record for this book
is available from the British Library

ISBN 0–632–03841–1

Library of Congress
Cataloging in Publication Data

Johnston, A. M.
    Equine medical disorders/
  A.M. Johnston.—2nd ed.
        p.   cm.
    (Library of veterinary practice)
    Includes bibliographical references
  (p.   ) and index.
    ISBN 0-632-03841-1
    1. Horses—Diseases.
    2. Horses—Wounds and injuries.
    I. Title II. Series.
  SF951.J64   1994
  636.1'0896—dc20

Contents

6   Internal parasites, 92

7   Skin diseases, 102

**8   Diseases of the
    musculoskeletal system, 117**

9   Cardiovascular system, 123

Preface to the second edition

The second edition follows the intention of the first, namely, to be of practical help to veterinary surgeons in practice and also to students.

This edition has a slightly larger format, with improved clarity in the layout of chapters and subsections. All chapters have been revised, some enlarged, and the sequence changed. New to this edition is a chapter on the cardiovascular system. There is improved discussion of neonatal problems, musculoskeletal and other diseases. The Notifiable Diseases section has been updated to include contagious equine metritis and equine viral arteritis, with reference made to the *Code of Practice for Control of Equine Reproductive Disease*, which is revised at regular intervals.

Note has been taken of the many helpful comments from clinical colleagues and the reviewers of the first edition, and these are reflected in this new edition. My clinical colleagues have again been most willing to give advice during the preparation of the second edition, and I am also grateful to Mrs Rosemary Forster for considerable help with its production.

Preface to the first edition

It is intended that this book will be of practical help to final year students and veterinary surgeons in general practice. As the book progressed a change in title, from the original *Infectious Diseases of the Horse*, was required by the inclusion of related non-infectious material.

Sections such as 'Orphan foal rearing' and 'Procedures which may aid diagnosis' have been included as the appropriate texts are seldom readily available to the practitioner in the field, when the information is most required.

The drug dosage information has been checked with the current data sheets but is not intended to replace this information, which may have been altered since preparation of the manuscript.

As a practical guide it is, on occasions, necessarily dogmatic, in particular with regard to the *reference values* given for laboratory tests and drug dosages. The clinician must at all times fully consider this information in relation to the clinical findings before making a decision on a diagnosis or treatment.

1 / Respiratory diseases

Diseases of the respiratory system probably account for the greatest number of clinical problems of any system of the horse. Coughing is a main sign; it results from respiratory disease and is a common reason for a veterinary consultation being requested. Studies of equine respiratory disease since the early 1970s indicate a very complex aetiology involving many viral agents and bacteria as well as a variety of host and management factors.

The evaluation of respiratory disease includes establishing:
1 Location – upper or lower respiratory tract;
2 Severity – degree of functional compromise;
3 Identification of causal agent(s).

This requires taking a very careful history, and a clinical examination with the possible use of diagnostic aids.

History
Age and breed of subject
Numbers of horses affected
Duration – acute (days) or chronic (weeks/months)
Signs seen by owner
Vaccinal status
Incidence of respiratory disease in the neighbourhood
Recent contacts or purchases
Environment (see diagram below)

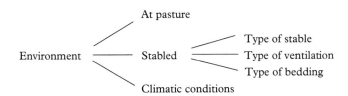

Clinical examination
Rate and character of breathing
Rectal temperature
Nasal discharge – volume and type
Cough – incidence and type
Lymph nodes – size and consistency
Percussion (see Fig. 1.1a)

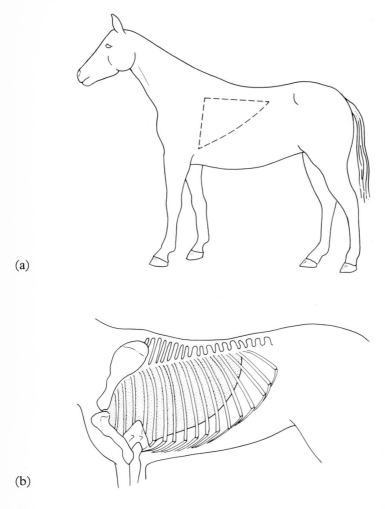

Fig. 1.1(a) Area of lung field as identified by percussion. **(b)** Schematic representation of area occupied by the left lung.

Ausculation (see Fig. 1.1b)
Effect of exercise

Aids to diagnosis
Haematology
Tracheal wash
Mucociliary clearance measurement
Fibreoptoscopic examination
Examination of faeces samples
Microbiology/virology/serology

Radiography
Response to treatment
Response to management changes

Aetiology
Viral infections
Bacterial infections
  (a) Primary
  (b) Secondary to viral infection
Allergies
Parasitic infections
Fungal infections
Aspiration pneumonia
  Injurious agents may gain access to the lungs by the airborne, the haematogenous or direct routes.

Resolution of changes
Rest
Antibacterial drugs
Anti-inflammatory drugs
Anthelmintics
Bronchodilators
Management changes

Viral respiratory disease

Most horse owners and trainers experience clinical respiratory disease in their horses each year and refer to it as 'the cough'. A more subtle 'poor performance' syndrome is also recognized when horses of known ability perform below par and are referred to as 'having the virus'. However, multiple infections of EHV, Rhinovirus 1 and 2, Picornavirus and adenovirus have been recognized and such mixed infections may be more important.

Equine influenza

Probably one of the most significant agents of respiratory disease in the horse occurs in epizootics and involves the myxovirus group of viruses. The following viral subtypes have been recorded:
* Myxovirus infection A/Equi 1
* Myxovirus infection A/Equi 2
Both affect the upper and lower respiratory tract with A/Equi 2, a more pneumotrophic virus, producing more severe clinical signs. In addition to the early viral subtypes of A/Equi 1 Prague (1956) and A/Equi 2 Miami

(1963), more recently A/Equi 2 Sussex and A/Equi 2 Suffolk virus strains have been isolated, the latter isolated during the United Kingdom's most recent major outbreak of equine flu. The antigenic drift which took place in 1979–81 produced variants of the Miami virus such as Solvalla '79, Fontainebleau '79, Kentucky '79 and others.

Clinical signs
Sudden onset
Frequent dry cough
Nasal discharge – serous but may become purulent if opportunist pathogens
    (mainly *Streptococcus zooepidemicus*) present
Fever – commonly 40°C (104°F) but up to 41°C (106°F)
Variable degree of dullness and anorexia
Submaxillary lymph nodes may be painful initially but show no obvious
    swelling
In foals a primary viral pneumonia can occur

Diagnosis
From history and clinical signs
Virus isolation using nasopharyngeal swabs which must be done early in the
    disease course
Serology with paired samples taken in the acute and convalescent phase. A
    four-fold rise in HI (haemagglutination inhibition test) titre provides
    confirmation

Differential diagnosis
Other viral or bacterial tract infections

Treatment
Symptomatic treatment with good nursing and hygiene. Affected and suspected in-contact horses should be isolated if possible.

The virus is shed for six days with an incubation period of five days.

In addition to respiratory disease the virus causes inflammatory changes in the myocardium and liver. It is essential that all work is stopped immediately and that there is a minimum of one month's complete rest after the disappearance of respiratory signs.

Prognosis
Good in uncomplicated cases where a marked improvement is seen in one week. Major secondary problems are:
- Bacterial rhinitis/pharyngitis
- Bacterial pneumonias

In foals, mortality can be high, in particular with A/Equi 2 virus when a primary viral pneumonia is usually fatal within four days of the onset of symptoms.

Prevention

Isolation is only practical where horses live in isolated circumstances with few outside contacts. A minimum period of 11 days, during which no new cases of influenza are identified, should elapse before a yard is considered clear for horses to leave or enter.

Vaccination is the only means of disease prevention and is currently required under Jockey Club Rules. Killed vaccines containing the commonly occurring A/Equi 1 and A/Equi 2 antigens are used. There is no cross-immunity between subtypes 1 and 2. Vaccines continue to include A/Equi 1 Prague, a strain which no longer appears to be circulating anywhere in the world. It is possible, by inclusion of A/Equi 2 Suffolk '89 strain, to provide either specific protection or cross-protection against the Miami and Miami-like viruses. The antibody response to the primary course of vaccination is about 6 months, with an age-related fall in detectable antibody level. The detectable antibody level of A/Equi 2 is less than A/Equi 1, with both falling more rapidly in young animals, in particular two- and three-year-old thoroughbreds in full training. The suggested annual booster vaccination is not sufficient, as immunity does not last a full year, only 6–9 months, unless a newer vaccine is used which is claimed to provide protection for 15 months.

N.B. Vaccination against equine influenza must not be regarded as protection against upper respiratory tract virus infections. A flu-like respiratory disease in a vaccinated animal may be due to:

1 Failure of the animal to respond to the vaccine.
2 Another virus which gives rise to similar clinical signs.
3 Different antigenic type of virus, or antigenic drift/shift.

Severe physical exercise, training or transportation are best avoided for 2–3 days following vaccination. Myocarditis or myositis can be sequelae if the horse is worked hard following vaccination.

Jockey Club Rules require the second injection in a primary course of flu vaccination to be given not less than 21 days and not more than 92 days after the first injection. The primary course in many horses will be given with a combined flu and tetanus vaccine. The minimum interval for such a combined vaccine is four weeks (see Chapter 13).

Equine herpes virus

Two viruses are involved:
- EHV-1 (Rhinopneumonitis)
- EHV-2 (Cytomegalovirus)

EHV-1 is of major importance and has two subtypes:

1 *Subtype 1 (known as EHV-1 and equine abortion virus)*
   Respiratory disease
   Abortion, stillbirth and neonatal death
   Posterior ataxia and paresis
2 *Subtype 2 (known as EHV-4 and Respiratory Herpes Strain)*
   Respiratory disease

Subtype 1 is common in the USA and was virtually unheard of in the UK until 1979, since when there has been an increasing number of reports of disease due to subtype 1. Outbreaks normally occur in autumn/winter, when large numbers of yearlings are brought together at sales and training yards.

EHV-1 is considered potentially more dangerous than EHV-4 as it can cause abortion storms, while EHV-4 causes only the occasional, isolated abortion. With both the infection starts with the respiratory system, but with EHV-1 it moves on to the foetus, in pregnant mares, or the brain and spinal cord in paralysis cases.

Isolation of EHV-1 from a competition or working horse merits serious consideration. The virus may invade the white cells and remain there for some weeks, which can compromise performance or ability to fight off other infections. The affected horse may also be a potential source of EHV-1 infection for breeding, or future breeding stock.

Respiratory form

The respiratory form (subtype 1 or 2) is usually seen in younger horses.

Lesions present include necrosis of the respiratory epithelium and lymph germinal centres which may be important in the development of secondary infection. Reinfection, or activation of latent infection, can lead to a sub-clinical infection which does not produce overt respiratory signs but does reduce the animal's performance.

Clinical signs

Cough, less pronounced than in equine influenza
Fever, up to 41°C (106°F)
Nasal discharge, serous becoming purulent
Variable degrees of dullness and anorexia
Submaxillary lymph nodes swollen

Diagnosis

From history and clinical signs
Haematology – leucopenia
Virus isolation from nasal swabs
Serology with paired samples taken in the acute and convalescent phases

Differential diagnosis
Other upper respiratory tract infections
Strangles

Treatment
Complete rest for at least three weeks
The use of antibacterials to control the secondary bacterial infection is
  frequently required and may be used in conjunction with bronchial
  mucolytics

Prognosis
A secondary rhinitis and pharyngitis frequently occur with a mucopurulent
nasal discharge and cough. These signs usually disappear in 1–3 weeks but
may persist for 1–2 months.

Persistent coughing may follow, without other clinical signs, and may
delay the horse's return to work. Complete rest, or only very light exercise,
for 2–3 weeks after the fever subsides is said to reduce the incidence of this
persistent coughing.

Neurological disease (subtype 1)
This EHV-1 myeloencephalopathy or paresis is seen in horses which have
previously been exposed to EHV-1 subtype 1 infection and where immunity
has waned and they have been reinfected by the same virus. This may lead to
an acute vasculitis with the end result of ischaemic lesions in the CNS.

Adults are usually affected and show signs within 12 days of exposure to
the virulent virus excreted by an aborting mare or an animal with respiratory
disease.

Clinical signs
Fever
Respiratory signs which may precede the CNS signs
Posterior ataxia or a non-specific hind leg lameness
Urinary incontinence
Flaccid vulval lips or penile prolapse
Recumbency, in severe cases

Diagnosis
Virus isolation from nasopharyngeal swabs which must be taken in the early
acute phase and sent to the laboratory in transport media. Serology with a
four-fold rise in titre is diagnostic. Samples are taken in the acute phase and
two weeks later. Another sample at six weeks may be required, depending on
the result; respiratory strains may take up to six weeks to show the four-fold
rise due to poor antibody response.

Treatment

Prevent the animal becoming recumbent or injuring itself, with the use of slings if necessary

Antibacterial therapy must be used if there is any evidence of secondary bacterial infection

Corticosteroids are of debatable value but if they are to be used it should be before the animal becomes ataxic

Prognosis

A guarded prognosis must be given.

Mares with incoordination or paresis may recover if abortion occurs or is induced in the early stages of the disease process.

Foals born near or at full term may be alive but are weak, frequently unable to suckle or stand and may be in severe respiratory distress. Bacterial infections and pneumonia frequently ensue and the foal dies in a few hours or within 3–4 days.

Prevention of EHV infection

Rapid diagnosis is important. Disperse and isolate horses in small groups, if possible, until a diagnosis of EHV is confirmed. All results of epizoological and virological studies of EHV indicate that the source of infection is another horse. It is also reasonable to assume that the carrier state exists and activation of latent infections due to 'stress' is an essential factor in maintaining the virus in the population.

Acquired immunity lasts up to 3–4 months after natural infection with little cross-infection between subtypes. There is a virally induced immunodeficiency in prenatally infected foals. Colostral antibodies from mares are present in the foal for three months. Reinfection has a much reduced rate of viral multiplication due to pre-existing acquired immunity.

Vaccines are available, but only poor, short-lived antibody levels are achieved.

Follow the code of practice established by the Thoroughbred Breeders' Association for studs where an EHV-1 abortion occurs.

EHV-2 infection

EHV-2 infection is of minor importance, with the virus found in the respiratory and genital tract of normal and abnormal horses. It has been linked with pharyngeal follicular hyperplasia.

In the adult there is a slight nasal discharge, no fever, an occasional cough and a period of poor performance. In foals there is a serous nasal discharge with no fever or malaise.

Rhinovirus

Recovered equine rhinoviruses are Rhinovirus type 1 and equine Rhinovirus type 2. Infection is common in young horses especially when brought together as two-year-olds in racing yards. Studies in British studs and training stables indicate that up to 25% of horses may have experienced infection before entering the training stable and approximately 30% of susceptible horses acquire infection during their first winter in training.

Clinical signs
Mild cough
Serous nasal discharge
Variable degrees of anorexia and depression
Lymph node enlargement common

Diagnosis
From history and clinical signs
Virus isolation using nasopharyngeal swabs
Serology using paired samples taken in the acute and convalescent phases

Differential diagnosis
Other upper respiratory tract infections, in particular those of viral origin.

Treatment
Usually there is a spontaneous improvement within 5–7 days.

Although the virus causes mild respiratory tract infections, there can be secondary bacterial infections which require antibacterial therapy.

Prognosis
Good for an uneventful recovery but the horse must not be worked while it has clinical signs of the viral infection.

Prevention
Rhinovirus 1 infection results in high antibody titres which are maintained for long periods and it is likely that immunity extends for life. No evidence of virus persistence has been found after a month; a carrier state is thus unlikely.

Inactivated vaccines can be produced without difficulty but the response is short-lived and frequent vaccinations would be required.

Rhinovirus II differs in that recovered horses continue to carry the virus for long periods. There is the potential for an ample reservoir of carriers to infect susceptible horses in large stables. Prevention of infection is difficult and following the introduction of a horse excreting the virus, Rhinovirus 2 infection will become enzootic in that group of horses.

Studies have shown decreasing antibody titres when the animals are at pasture and increasing titres during periods of housing.

No vaccine is available.

Adenovirus

Adenovirus infections are extremely common in the horse with many of the infections occurring in the first year of life.

Clinical signs

1   A mild upper respiratory tract infection accompanied by soft faeces or a mild, transient diarrhoea.

2   A true viral pneumonia in immunodeficient, usually Arabian, foals (see Chapter 5).

Diagnosis

From suggestive clinical signs

Haematology – a severe absolute lymphopenia with a progressive reduction of total leucocytes

Finding intranuclear inclusions in smears of conjunctival or nasal epithelium

Post-mortem examination

Macroscopic lesions found include:

- Mucopurulent exudate in the upper respiratory tract
- Bronchopneumonia with atelectasis
- Ulceration of the oral mucosa
- Ulceration of the gut mucosa with atrophy of the lymph nodes

Treatment

Control of secondary bacterial or fungal infections is essential

Supportive therapy with electrolyte and glucose solutions, and antidiarrhoeal products

Possible use of whole blood, plasma or serum transfusion from a dam with high antibody levels

Corticosteroids are contraindicated (as the lymphopoietic system is depressed)

Prognosis

Morbidity is 10% and mortality approaches 100% of affected foals.

Prevention

Acquired immunity is poor and reinfection in a clinical or subclinical form is possible with as little as 3–4 months between episodes

No vaccine is available

At risk foals should have a clean, warm, dry, dust-free environment and be
    fed clean grass, hay and dust-free concentrate mixtures or pelleted feed

Picornavirus 4442/75

Subclinical infection with this virus is most common. Horses experimentally
infected with the virus intranasally did not show fever, leucopenia or
respiratory signs. Foals exposed to the virus may show signs some weeks after
weaning but this has not definitely been shown to be due to 4442/75 virus.

Summary

The majority of viral infections remain uncomplicated. A suggested scheme
for treating a horse with a runny nose/cough is as follows:
- No work for one month
- Nasal swabs and/or blood should be taken to identify the cause
- Antipyretic drugs are valuable in improving the horse's attitude and
appetite
- Antibiotic therapy, if considered necessary, for a minimum of three days
prophylactically or five days therapeutically
- Mucolytics, e.g. Sputolosin (Boehringer Ingelheim Ltd)
- Bronchodilators – clenbuterol hydrochloride

Bacterial respiratory disease

The streptococci of Lancefield Group C are important causes of bacterial
respiratory disease, in particular *Streptococcus equi* and *Streptococcus zooepidemicus*. Both produce suppurative infections of the horse and either may
result in the development of purpura haemorrhagica.

Results of a study indicate that *Streptococcus pneumoniae* is carried by
many horses in training yards. On available evidence, it appears that *S.
pneumoniae* can play an important role in respiratory disease. Other bacteria,
e.g. *Escherichia coli*, staphylococci, *Klebsiella* are usually associated with a
bacteraemia.

S. zooepidemicus, *S. equi*, *E. coli*, *Staphylococcus aureus* and *Pseudomonas*
spp. are potential pathogens in viral respiratory disease.

Bacterial pneumonia

The role of bacteria as primary agents of pneumonia in the horse is difficult
to assess. The condition has multiple causes including infectious agents and
environmental factors.

Pathogens involved are usually organisms ubiquitous to the environment and reach the lower respiratory tract by:
- Inhalation – aerosol
- Haematogenous spread, e.g. *Klebsiella* or *Salmonella*
- Transport of the organism by a migrating parasite - *Rhodococcus equi* from the gut

The organisms involved include:
- Streptococci (most commonly *S. zooepidemicus*)
- *Pasteurella* or *Actinobacillus* (frequently accompany streptococci)
- *R. equi* – see Chapter 5
- Staphylococci
- *Klebsiella*
- *Salmonella*
- *E. coli*
- *Pseudomonas*

History
In conjunction with a systemic disease, e.g. *E. coli* or *Salmonella*
As a sequel to a disease, e g. upper respiratory tract (URT) viral infection
Debility
Stress

Clinical signs
Elevated temperature and pulse rate
Elevated respiratory rate with laboured or difficult breathing in severe cases
Cyanosis of mucous membranes – variable
Moist cough with or without nasal discharge
Depression, lethargy, anorexia – variable depending on severity
Abnormal lung sounds – moist rales early and dry rales with pleural friction sounds later which will be absent over areas of consolidation
Fluid line – determine by percussion and lack of lung sounds over the whole area on auscultation (see Fig. 1.1a)

Diagnosis
History with clinical findings
Haematology – assess systemic response
Tracheal wash – enables identification of causal organisms at an early stage by direct smear and culture followed by antibiotic sensitivity
Radiography – evaluation of abscessation and confirm presence of a fluid line and its limits
Thoracocentesis if fluid line is present

Differential diagnosis
Pneumothorax, haemothorax or hydrothorax
A primary pleurisy

Treatment
Antibiotics – penicillin is probably best until sensitivity results are known, or trimethoprim/sulphonamide combination
Rest in clean, dry, dust-free environment
Bronchodilators and/or mucolytics
Corticosteroids – if it is considered that oedema and congestion produced by the acute inflammation are killing the horse faster than the bacteria, one dose of corticosteroid may be helpful (with antibiotics)
Oxygen

The response to treatment must be assessed at regular intervals and the therapy continued for some time after signs have resolved.

Prognosis
Must always be guarded as it depends on the amount of residual and permanent lung damage. There may also be the requirement for prolonged therapy, with chronic bronchitis and emphysema possible sequelae. The earlier treatment is instituted in acute cases, the more favourable the prognosis. If the resting respiratory rate stays high the prognosis is poor.

Chronic bronchitis

Chronic bronchitis and bronchiolitis are common in the horse and are frequently a sequel to respiratory tract infections. Bacteria are potentially causative agents and streptococci, staphylococci, *E. coli* and *Pseudomonas* can be isolated from the exudates.

Clinical signs
Cough
Expiratory dyspnoea
Reduced exertional capability
Dry rales on auscultation of ventral lung fields
Haematology – leucocytosis
Tracheal wash – presence of macrophages and neutrophils

Treatment
Antibiotics – penicillins or sulphonamides are often successful
Clean, dust-free environment
Mucolytic or expectorant drugs may be of benefit

Prognosis

Depends on the response to treatment and presence or absence of alveolar emphysema. There is frequently a history of previous respiratory disease or allergic reaction. The prognosis for a full recovery must be guarded until the initial response to therapy is known and sufficient time has elapsed without a recurrence of the signs.

Strangles – *Streptococcus equi* infection

Traditionally, strangles occurred in young horses of three months to three years of age, as older horses had been exposed to earlier epizootics. Such epizootics are now rare and the infection may be seen in horses of all ages. The mode of infection can be by inhalation or orally.

Horses will exhibit signs of disease 2–6 days after the infection but the incubation period can be ten days at the start of an outbreak.

Clinical signs

Clinical signs are mainly due to the localization of the organism in the URT and associated lymph nodes, but affected animals are bacteraemic in the first 2–3 days after infection.

Early phase

Frequently bacteraemic
Depression and anorexia
Fever 38–39.5°C (100.5–103°F)
Slight submaxillary lymph node enlargement
Slight ocular and nasal discharge
Slight cough

Later phase

Prominent cough and purulent nasal discharge
Marked depression, anorexia and dysphagia
Fever 39.5–41°C (103–106°F)
Submaxillary lymph nodes obviously enlarged

In the initial stage of infection the streptococcus produces abscesses in the lymphoid follicles of the pharyngeal mucosa. At this stage the horse is reluctant to swallow due to the pain. These abscesses mature and drain quickly with infection spreading to the pharyngeal and submaxillary lymph nodes.

Diagnosis

From suggestive clinical signs
Haematology – neutrophilia
Bacterial culture

Treatment

Affected horses should not be worked

Antibiotic therapy, in particular procaine penicillin in large doses for at least
five days

Non-steroidal anti-inflammatory drugs may reduce the pain and improve
appetite

If reluctant to feed give soft, sloppy foods

Remove purulent discharges with non-irritating antiseptic solution

Warm compresses on the abscess

If the airway is obstructed a tracheostomy will be required

Prognosis

In untreated cases the abscessed lymph nodes mature, rupture and drain
within two weeks with a rapid clinical improvement. Continued fever and
depression indicates the involvement of other sites and is called 'bastard
strangles' but the incidence of this is usually low.

If the infection is diagnosed in the early phase then antibiotic treatment is
indicated, as it can stop the dissemination of the streptococci to internal sites
and prevent localization in the URT or lymph nodes. In the later phase it is
theoretically possible that antibiotic therapy may delay or prevent abscess
maturation. In such cases antibiotic therapy may be withheld until abscesses
have ruptured.

Prevention

Isolate affected animals with strict hygiene control of all persons and utensils
in contact. Spread can be by direct or indirect contact, thus disinfection of
all tack, especially the head collar and grooming equipment, which should
be kept separate, must be done thoroughly.

Any swabs or material used to clean discharges should be burnt.

Stables housing clinical cases or possible clinical cases should be cleaned
and disinfected after the horses have recovered. All new, in particular
yearling, horses brought into the yard should be isolated for three weeks if
possible.

Internal abscessation

Abscesses can be found within either the thoracic or abdominal cavities and
may result in the death of the horse. They may occur as a sequel to:

- Bacteraemia, e.g. strangles
- Cryptococcal pneumonia
- Penetrating wounds including foreign body penetration of gut wall
- Castration or abdominal surgery
- Rectal tears and perforations

Clinical signs
Anorexia
Weight loss
Intermittent fever
Intermittent colic
Depression – variable

Diagnosis
History most important
Haematology – leucocytosis (10 000–60 000 total white blood cells (WBC))
    with a shift to the left
Blood chemistry – hypergammaglobulinaemia with hypoalbuminaemia and
    lowered albumin/globulin ratio
Increased plasma fibrinogen (>400 mg/dl) in inflammatory conditions rising
    to >1000 mg/dl in chronic, active conditions

Thoracic abscesses
Percussion – may detect fluid line but unlikely to detect abscess
Thoracocentesis – may be of value if exudate present in the pleural space
    (N. B. always do both sides of the chest)
Radiography – is a valuable aid to diagnosis when practicable, e.g. with foals
    or if an X-ray machine of sufficient power is available for adult horses
Any abscess must be large enough and have a well-developed capsule to be
    radiographically opaque

Abdominal abscesses
Rectal examination – 50% of abdominal abscesses have palpable mass
    and/or pain in the splenic and renal areas
Paracentesis – 50% of the cases give evidence of peritonitis,
    i.e. S.G.> 1.017
    Protein > 25 g/l
    WBC > 10 000 cells
    Fibrinogen – large amounts

Differential diagnosis
Disseminated 'strangles'
Neoplasia

Treatment
Long term antibiotic therapy. When the causal organism is unknown, the
most efficacious antibiotic is procaine penicillin at a dose of 20 million units
daily. The trimethoprim/sulphonamide combinations may have a role in
these cases if there does not appear to be a response to the penicillin therapy.

Prognosis

A very guarded prognosis must be given. Affected horses usually have a prolonged period of insidious wasting, low-grade fever and slight leucocytosis: should this picture continue after a reasonable period of therapy, the prognosis must be considered hopeless. Long term, high dose level antibiotic therapy may precipitate complications such as salmonellosis or colitis X.

Prevention

It is possible to speculate that inadequate antibiotic therapy may have a role to play in the development of internal abscesses. If antibiotic therapy is instituted for respiratory disease or lymphoid abscessation it should be continued, at therapeutic levels, until after the cessation of clinical signs.

Allergic respiratory disease

This is a common cause of chronic respiratory disease in the adult horse. Traditionally, severely affected animals were recognized by their poor exercise tolerance and pronounced expiratory effort at rest. Although also known as 'broken wind', 'heaves' or 'chronic alveolar emphysema', it is best referred to as obstructive pulmonary disease (OPD) or small airway disease. It is normally a chronic non-febrile disease but cases do seem to follow acute febrile respiratory tract infections, in particular those with a viral component, which sensitizes the horse.

The inhaled allergens have two main effects:
1 Direct stimulation of irritant receptors in the larynx and trachea.
2 Induction of the allergic response.

Clinical signs

May be intermittent with their presence or absence dependent on exposure to the allergen. The clinical signs reflect an increase in airway resistance due to a decrease in airway size and this produces:
1 Smooth muscle spasm.
2 Inflammatory response around the airways.
3 Excessive mucus within the airways.
This is reflected in an increased rate and depth of respiration and coughing: much of the mucus coughed is swallowed.

Mild cases
Chronic cough
Normal respiratory rate and character
Normal lung sounds
Possible serous nasal discharge

Moderately severe cases
Chronic cough
Increased respiratory rate and effort
Harsh lung sounds with crackles
Nasal discharge may be present
Unable to sustain work without respiratory distress

Severe cases
Chronic cough
Very rapid respiratory rate (20–40+ per minute)
Markedly increased effort with double expiratory movement
'Heave' line present
Unable to do work without becoming breathless
Weight loss

Diagnostic aids
Endoscopy – excessive tracheal mucus
Tracheal wash – sterile, many neutrophils present
Haematology – usually normal
Faecal samples – to eliminate possible lungworm infection
Response to a dust-free environment for at least four days
Response to therapeutic drugs
Radiography – very difficult to interpret
Change in intrapleural pressure – normal 4 mmHg; affected 6 mmHg or
    more
Arterial oxygen tension – normal 90 mmHg; affected 82 mmHg or less

Diagnosis
This presents no problem in moderate to severe cases. Any horse with a
respiratory rate in excess of 20 breaths per minute with increased effort, with
no evidence of infectious respiratory disease, will almost certainly be OPD.
    Other cases rely on:
- history
- clinical signs
- diagnostic aids
- management

Differential diagnosis
Colic – in very acute cases, apart from the above findings, the horse sweats, is
    uncomfortable and may be presented as a colic
Lungworm
Pneumonia

Treatment
Specific bronchodilator – clenbuterol hydrochloride

Inhibit/prevent mast cell degranulation – sodium cromoglycate (or corticosteroids). The former is preferred and should be given when the OPD is asymptomatic, giving 3–4 weeks protection from a 4-day course of treatment

Remove allergen – the most effective measure achieved by the following methods:

1 Stable management of the highest standard. If possible, keep the horse out of doors for as much of the year as possible. When stabled, keep the horses away when boxes are being mucked out, and as far away as possible from the dung heap.

2 Bedding should be paper, shavings, peat or damped straw, with dust kept to a minimum.

3 Feed should be best hay damped or preferably hosed, complete cubed horse food or other conserved grass products, e.g. Horsehage.

Prognosis
The lung changes are considered to be reversible until alveolar breakdown takes place. As most cases do not develop significant alveolar emphysema until severely affected, the prognosis is good provided appropriate treatment is instigated and maintained.

Each exposure to the dust/allergen to which the horse is sensitized will produce a more severe response. The severity of the signs therefore tends to increase with each succeeding year.

An OPD horse can be asymptomatic and produce a response varying from mild to acutely symptomatic depending on the individual challenge. The prognosis is therefore very dependent on the ability or willingness of the owner to achieve a permanent asymptomatic OPD state.

Prevention
All horses and ponies can develop allergic respiratory disease. It is essential that stable management is of the highest standard for all, but especially for young horses that could become sensitized before they even start to fulfil the purpose for which they were bred or purchased.

Chemotherapy should be looked on as a means of controlling acute bouts, but not for long-term use.

Parasitic respiratory disease

Mature horse – *Dictyocaulus arnfieldi*
Dictyocaulus arnfieldi produces a parasitic bronchitis

Clinical signs

Persistent cough for months, or even longer than one year

Possible increased respiratory rate with adventitious lung sounds which may diminish in intensity

Non-progressive syndrome

Diagnosis

A very carefully taken history is essential

Can be very difficult on clinical signs alone and frequently is by a satisfactory reponse to specific anthelmintic therapy

Haematology – may show an eosinophilia

Faecal examinations – positive results can be interpreted with more confidence than negative ones

Tracheal wash – eosinophils and, on occasion, *Dictyocaulus* larvae; no bacteria

Treatment

Anthelmintics are known to be effective against *Dictyocaulus*, which may acquire a different dose rate from that for routine worm control, e.g. fenbendazole at 15 mg/kg bodyweight; thiabendazole at 440 mg/kg, repeated at 48 hours; ivermectin 200 mg/kg.

Prognosis

A full recovery is made following anthelmintic treatment but the horse may become infected again. Infections in horses may be more common than the incidence of respiratory disease indicates, with most horses not developing patent infections. Shared grazing with donkeys, which have a much higher incidence of *Dictyocaulus* infection and develop patent infection in a high percentage of affected animals, is a likely source of infection.

Foals – *Parascaris equorum*: see Chapter 6.

Fungal respiratory infection

Fungal pneumonia in horses is rare despite the horse's inevitable exposure to fungal spores. Cases of pneumonia due to *Aspergillus* species and *Cryptococcus neoformans* have been recorded. Nasal aspergillosis has also been reported, more frequently associated with paranasal sinusitis.

Clinical signs

Nasal discharge – foul-smelling, scanty (unilateral)

Chronic cough

Weight loss

Possible spread of fungal infection to other systems, in particular uterine involvement and abortion

Post-mortem examination

Grey nodules, in variable numbers over all lung areas, 1–10 mm in diameter, surrounded by granulomatous reaction

Culture of causal fungus may be possible

Diagnosis

Extremely difficult from clinical examination alone

Tracheal aspiration – fungal hyphae may be found, but they can also be found in samples taken from clinically normal horses in dusty barns

Radiography – quite helpful, as the lungs appear diffuse greyish on the radiograph due to the large number of small nodules

Serology – only indicates the presence of recent infection and not the presence of active disease

Treatment

Nystatin can be tried

Natamycin in an aerosol form daily for six weeks has been used with some success in human fungal respiratory infections

Prognosis

Poor.

Cryptococcal respiratory infection

Most common species is *Cryptococcus neoformans*. Produces either diffuse and multiple lesions with bilateral involvement or localized lesions in one lung. May present as meningitis or as nasal granulomas.

Diagnosis

The lesions can show as well-defined, round, soft tissue masses on radiographs of the chest

Yeast cells may be found on tracheal aspirate but may only be isolated in some 20% of cases

Treatment and prognosis

Poor prognosis. Treatment with amphotericin B has been used in humans and small animals with some success but without success in horses. In most cases treatment is not attempted.

N.B. Thought to be related in humans to reduced immune status. If suspected, do not use corticosteroids.

Aspiration pneumonia

Aspiration pneumonia is an uncommon but very severe condition when present. It may be due to:
- Regurgitation of food material – in oesophageal obstruction
- Pharyngeal paresis or paralysis
- Structural abnormality – cleft palate in a foal
- Induced
  intrapulmonary administration of medication, e.g. wormers
  milk inhalation in fostered foals
  partial drowning

Clinical signs
As for severe respiratory illness
Clinical signs of principal cause – e.g. 'choke' (milk or wormer material coming down nose)

Diagnosis
Clinical signs
Tracheal wash – confirmation of presence of foreign material

Treatment
Antibacterial therapy
Steroids in large doses to limit the inflammatory response to irritating chemicals
Try suction, if necessary, following tracheotomy
Food and water by stomach tube if necessary
Cross-tie horse with head down

Prognosis
Depends on the quantity and type of material inhaled
Initially give a very guarded prognosis and be prepared to revise it following subsequent examinations
If the cause is choke, which is resolved, the lungs do a remarkable job of resolving the problem
If the cause is wormers, the prognosis is poor and worse if food material is inhaled

Smoke inhalation injury

Both heat and toxic gases cause damage to the respiratory tract. The main mechanisms are direct thermal injury of the upper airway and chemical injury of the tracheo-bronchial airway and pulmonary parenchyma. Carbon monoxide may cause poisoning at the time of, or shortly after, exposure. Toxic gases can be absorbed onto soot particles and carried down into the lungs. Heat produces erythema, oedema and ulceration.

Noxious gases include sulphur, hydrocyanic acid, nitrous oxides, toxic gases from plastics. The onset of injury is rapid if the gases are highly water-soluble. Combination with water will form corrosive acids. Aldehydes denature protein and can cause pulmonary oedema.

Treatment
Provide patent airway - tracheostomy may be necessary
Decrease oedema - frusemide
Decrease bronchoconstriction with bronchodilators
Prevent oedema and bronchoconstriction - non-steroidal anti-inflammatory drugs
Provide ventilatory support - humidified oxygen
Intravenous fluids for horses which are also burned require monitoring for pulmonary oedema

Pleuritis and pleural effusions

Pleuritis is commonly associated with acute or chronic pneumonia or lung abscesses and best referred to as pleuropneumonia. The 'dry' stage, with an exudate of lymph, fibrin and cellular elements, may progress to the effusive stage with fluid accumulation, from serum exudation, in the pleural cavity.
Pleural effusion is not common in the horse. Normal, clear, serous fluid is present which will yield up to 8 ml on thoracocentesis.

N.B. The pleural cavities frequently communicate with one another as the posterior mediastinum is very delicate.

Clinical signs
Vary in proportion to the amount of pleural fluid
Pain
Respiratory rate and pattern altered with eventual 'distress' where large quantities are present
Subacute or chronic cases - weight loss, anorexia, exercise intolerance, recurrent pneumonia
Fever may be recurrent or constant
Subcutaneous oedema of sternal/pectoral regions and limbs in long-standing cases.

Diagnosis
Reduced or absent lung sounds on ventral thorax. Dorsal lung sounds may be normal

Heart sounds heard over a greater area
Fluid line detected by percussion

Aids to diagnosis
Radiography to confirm presence of an effusion
Ultrasonography to demonstrate pleural fluid, pleural adhesions and
    pulmonary consolidation
Thoracocentesis (from both sides of the chest) with submission of the fluid
    for cytological examination and bacterial culture

Treatment
Removal of fluid – remove enough fluid to relieve dyspnoea and then the
    remainder over 24 hours. Indwelling chest tubes are recommended
    which have been tunnelled subcutaneously before insertion into thoracic
    cavity and attached to a one-way valve.
    N.B. Rapid removal of large amounts of fluid may induce hypovolaemic
    crisis, hypoxaemia and hypoproteinaemia.
Appropriate antibiotic therapy – initially broad spectrum until results of
    bacterial culture known
Analgesia and anti-inflammatory drugs, e.g. flunixin or opiates if the pain is
    severe
General supportive therapy

Prognosis
Initially best decided when the results of radiography and ultrasonography,
following removal of the thoracic fluid, have been considered, along with the
laboratory findings on the fluid. Treatment is usually attempted in cases
secondary to pneumonia or lung abscesses.
    Very poor prognosis is associated with systemic problems.

Haemothorax

Seen with trauma when vessels are ruptured, ribs fractured with possible
damage to the lung parenchyma. May also be present with clotting disorders.

Diagnosis
Based on clinical examination and thoracocentesis
Radiographs and ultrasonography are also very helpful

Treatment
Treat the underlying cause. May be necessary to remove piece of fractured
    rib

Remove any blood, and air if there is a pneumothorax, which may have to be
   repeated
Antibiotic cover and analgesics as necessary

Prognosis
Depends on underlying cause. Uncomplicated trauma responds well.
Poor prognosis if clotting disorders or neoplasia unless clotting disorder is
   secondary to the use of drugs which can be stopped.

Pneumothorax

Usually associated with trauma but can follow pneumonia.

Clinical signs
May include:
- evidence of a wound
- subcutaneous oedema
- increased respiratory rate/dyspnoea
- absence of normal lung sounds (dorsal thorax)
- increased resonance on percussion.

Diagnosis
From clinical signs
Air aspirated from pneumothorax by percutaneous puncture
Radiography

Treatment
Following trauma, occlude wound immediately with bulky sterile dressing
Close wound with chest tube inserted for decompression
Gradual aspiration of air to re-establish negative pressure
Antibiotics
Ensure any foreign material that could migrate into pleural cavity is removed
   N.B. It is possible to debride wound and suture appropriately later when
   horse is stabilized (as is the case for general anaesthesia)
Locate and stabilize any fractured ribs to prevent further damage
With pneumothorax from lung problems, fibrinous adhesions usually
   localize the leak and the pneumothorax does not become generalized
Treat the underlying cause of the primary problem

Pulmonary oedema

A life-threatening complication of primary diseases such as bacterial and viral
infections, toxins, endotoxic shock, disseminated intravascular coagulation

(DIC), anaphylaxis. Pulmonary oedema may recur in acute renal failure and be enhanced by too-rapid administration of intravenous fluids when there is increased microvascular permeability.

Clinical signs
Shallow, rapid respiration
May be dyspnoea
Crackles (moist), possible wheeze
Fluid may drip from nostrils (clear/yellow/pink-tinged)
Tracheal frothing

Diagnosis
From clinical signs
Radiographic findings non-specific, but there can be increased prominence
    of vessels and a hazy reticular or lattice pattern.

Treatment
Intranasal oxygen in severe cases
Diuretics – e.g. frusemide 0.5–1.0 mg/kg i.v.
Bronchodilators, e.g. clenbuterol
Stop intravenous fluid therapy
Steroids – to decrease capillary permeability with antibiotic therapy.
Whole blood or colloid solutions i.v. *very slowly*. Plasma may be safer than
    other colloid solutions.
Heparin if DIC present – 25–100 iu/kg/i.v.
Analgesia/anxiety relief – morphine-type drugs

Exercise-induced pulmonary haemorrhage

Haemorrhage from the lungs occurs in a large proportion of horses during racing. The appearance of blood at the nostrils, known as 'epistaxis' or 'bleeding' is seen in fewer than 10% of horses with exercise-induced pulmonary haemorrhage (EIPH). Small airway disease has been proposed as a factor predisposing to EIPH. The incidence increases with age.

Diagnosis
Examination by endoscopy of the tracheobronchial airway for the presence
    of blood
Check for poor or impaired performance or slowing or stopping, with
    greater swallowing, 'gurgling', 'choking' and/or coughing after exercise
The presence of macrophages containing haemosiderin help to confirm that
    a horse has had a previous EIPH
Unless co-existing disease is present, haematology and blood chemistry
    changes are not found

Treatment and prevention

A large number of 'treatments' are in use, with little evidence to allow their efficacy to be evaluated.

- Rest.
- Attention must be given to providing an environment free from dust and pathogens, to avoid small airway disease.
- Frusemide (0.3–0.6 mg/kg) is probably the most commonly used medication to prevent EIPH. It has not been shown to stop EIPH but has reduced the EIPH score.

Prognosis

While rest for 3–6 months will help some horses, most continue to experience EIPH when they return to competitive exercise. *Post-mortem* studies of retired horses from riding schools suggest that lesions take a long time to heal.

Purpura haemorrhagica

Purpura haemorrhagica may be a sequel to infectious disease, in particular β-haemolytic streptococcal infections. These are usually, but not restricted to, respiratory tract infections within the last month or so. The condition tends to appear either at the end of the acute phase or at the commencement of the convalescent phase.

The cause of the disease is not known but is thought to be a hypersensitivity reaction where antibody–antigen complexes adhere to and damage the capillary walls. The capillary wall endothelium is damaged allowing protein and blood loss.

History

Strangles

Viral URTdisease with or without secondary streptococcal infection

Streptococcal pneumonia

Administration of autogenous β-haemolytic streptococcal vaccine

There may be no history of clinical infection or any such infection may not have been noticed

Clinical signs

There is a considerable variation in the severity of clinical signs

Mild form

Muscle stiffness with the horse reluctant or unable to walk or move its neck

Temperature normal

Pulse normal

Respiratory rate normal (but may be at the upper end of the normal range)
Urticarial type lesions, which vary in size, on parts of the body
There may be slight oedema in legs, ventral abdomen and prepuce
No alteration in total RBC number

Severe form
Pronounced oedema, which may have appeared initially and become
    progressively more severe – usually head and legs first
Legs swell, with oedematous areas well-defined, and may exude serum, in
    particular over the joints
Petechial haemorrhages on the visible mucous membranes, tongue and
    vaginal mucosa
Nasal mucosa becomes congested and the oedema of the head develops
Variable degree of respiratory distress from involvement of the respiratory
    passages, pulmonary oedema or pulmonary haemorrhage
Temperature elevated up to 40.5°C (105°F) if secondary infection

Diagnosis
History
Clinical signs
Haematology – severe form – fall in total red blood cell count (RBC) to 3–4
    million/ml; fall in packed cell volume (PCV); haemoglobin decreases to
    7–8 g/ml; leucocytosis with a neutrophilia within 2–3 days. Often pla-
    telets normal, as are clotting times

Differential diagnosis
Acute laminitis in particular with mild form
Azoturia or 'tying up'
Chronic anthrax
Viral arteritis
Equine infectious anaemia
Idiopathic thrombocytopenic purpura – platelet count is down to 33 000/ml
    and in purpura haemorrhagica there is a normal platelet count

Post-mortem findings
Subcutaneous oedema
Increased amount of peritoneal fluid
Visible haemorrhages on all surfaces
Histopathologically – haemorrhage and oedema of muscle and lungs

Treatment
Corticosteroids initially given parenterally by the intravenous or intramus-
    cular route. If corticosteroid therapy is to be continued over a prolonged

period, the use of prednisolone tablets given orally, crushed in the food, should be considered, at a 0.04–0.1 mg/kg dose daily, with decrease over several weeks

Antibiotics, with penicillin the drug of first choice

Tracheotomy if there is respiratory distress

Blood transfusion may be necessary if the PCV < 15%

Good nursing care is essential – deep bedding, fresh water and palatable food. The legs should be bandaged with adequate cotton wool or gamgee and the horse given controlled walking exercise if possible

Prognosis

A grave prognosis should always be given. The mortality rate is variable and depends on the severity of the case, treatment, the standard of care and attention during the illness and at which stage of the disease process treatment was commenced

A mortality rate of 50% is possible with the severe form

Mild cases recover in 7–10 days

Severe cases can require up to 2–3 months to complete the recovery if skin necrosis is present. The oedema recedes over 2–4 weeks

2/Diseases of the alimentary tract

Diarrhoea in adult horses

Diarrhoea in the adult horse may not require veterinary attention as the horse may recover on its own in a few days.

Aetiology

Acute diarrhoea
Salmonellosis
Equine intestinal clostridiosis
Colitis X
Poisonings
Unknown aetiology

Chronic diarrhoea
Parasitic
    mixed strongyle infections
    Eimeria leuckarti infection
    trichomoniasis
Chronic salmonellosis
Antibiotic associated diarrhoea
Neoplasia
Malabsorption syndrome and granulomatous bowel disease
Undetermined cause

Clinical examination

Rectal temperature
Pulse – rate and character
Body condition – weight loss/dehydration
Faeces – volume, consistency, presence or absence of blood and epithelium
Auscultation – assessment of degree of hyper-hypomotility of gut and presence of tympany
Teeth – ensure that proper mastication of food can take place

Aids to diagnosis

Haematology
Blood chemistry
Faecal examination – microbiological, parasitological

Response to treatment
Response to management changes

Salmonellosis

Clinical disease typically affects individual stressed or debilitated animals. Occasionally outbreaks are recorded where grossly contaminated food or water is given to a group, or there is a common debilitating factor, e.g. internal parasitism. A proportion of clinically normal horses are carriers and shed the organisms either continuously or intermittently in their faeces. Surveys indicate that as many as one horse in five can be a carrier, with the organism most commonly in the large bowel and associated lymph nodes. (See Fig. 2.1.)

Peracute, acute, chronic and atypical syndromes are recognized.

Aetiology

Over 40 *Salmonella* serotypes have been isolated from horses, of which 75% were *S. typhimurium*. Other common serotypes are *S. enteritidis*, *S. newport*, *S. heidelberg* and *S. dublin*.

Peracute salmonellosis

This is seen mainly in foals.

Clinical signs

Sudden onset of septicaemia with enteric involvement
Fever of 40–41°C (104–106°F)
Depression, anorexia, weakness
Elevated heart rate with a weak pulse
Elevated respiratory rate

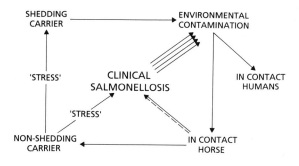

Fig. 2.1 Carriers of clinical salmonellosis.

Cyanotic mucous membranes with petechiation
Diarrhoea and abdominal pain common
Blood and epithelium in faeces uncommon
Dehydration and electrolyte imbalance rapidly develop

Aids to diagnosis
Haematology – very marked leucopenia (total white blood cells (WBC)
    2000/ml) due to neutropenia with degenerative left shift early in the
    course of the disease
Blood chemistry – rapid development of hypoalbuminaemia, fall in serum
    sodium and acidosis

Prognosis
The course of the disease is short, with the majority of animals dying within 72
hours, following dehydration, electrolyte imbalance and circulatory collapse.

Acute salmonellosis
This is mostly seen in adults.

Clinical signs
Sudden onset
Fever of 40–41.1°C (104–106°F) may be the first sign
Diarrhoea is possibly one of the first signs, with mild abdominal pain, but
    may not develop until day six in some cases
Elevated heart rate with a weak pulse
Elevated respiratory rate
Depression, anorexia, weakness
A terminal septicaemia may follow in many cases with marked dehydration,
    electrolyte imbalance and circulatory collapse

Aids to diagnosis
Haematology – early leucopenia (total WBC 1500–2000/ml) due to a
    neutropenia with degenerative shift to the left. This in itself is very
    suggestive of salmonellosis. There follows a neutrophilia with regen-
    erative left shift
Blood chemistry – rapid development of hypoalbuminaemia, less rapid
    development of hyponatraemia

Prognosis
Although the clinical signs are very similar to the peracute syndrome the
    horse tends to live longer, up to three weeks, and some may survive
Young foals affected die in 2–3 days whilst older foals may survive for up to
    ten days

Survivors may become:
    total recoveries and non-carriers
    asymptomatic carriers with no shedding
    asymptomatic carriers with intermittent or continuous shedding
    chronic cases

Chronic salmonellosis
This may present as a primary condition or as a sequel to acute salmonellosis.

Clinical signs
Thought to occur as a sequel to severe changes in the bowel wall
Soft faeces with bouts of diarrhoea
Persistent weight loss
Fever may be present
Anorexia may be present

Aids to diagnosis
Microbiological examination of faecal samples is most unrewarding with
    only very occasional samples yielding *Salmonella* organisms
Haematology – primary neutropenia with degenerative left shift followed by
    a neutrophilia and regenerative left shift

Prognosis
Symptoms may be present for weeks or months and the horse ultimately may
die or be destroyed.

Atypical salmonellosis
The stress of transport, participation in competitive events or being taken to
a veterinary centre for surgical or other procedures may trigger off a case of
asymptomatic salmonellosis (or asymptomatic shedding).

Clinical signs
Fever 39.4–41.1°C (103–106°F)
Anorexia
Depression
Mild abdominal pain
Soft faeces

Aids to diagnosis
Haematology – primary neutropenia with degenerative left shift followed by
    a neutrophilia with regenerative left shift
Microbiological examination – *Salmonella* organisms will be found in the

faeces for one or two days but organisms can be present for up to seven days

Prognosis
There is a spontaneous return to clinical normality in 3–7 days.

Diagnosis of salmonellosis
A provisional diagnosis has to be made on clinical signs supported by an initial, significant, neutropenia with a degenerative left shift as faecal culture takes a minimum of 2–3 days. Positive faecal cultures are most readily obtained from animals in the acute stage, with negative results difficult to interpret as intermittent excretion may occur.

Serology is of little value in the diagnosis of clinical cases.

Treatment
Fluids and electrolytes are essential. For accurate treatment electrolyte and acid/base evaluations should be carried out as there is a wide variation in fluid loss and intake between individual cases.

If there is a marked hypoalbuminaemia, the use of blood, plasma or plasma volume expander may be necessary.

Horses in shock with poor hepatic function may be unable to utilize bicarbonate. Bicarbonate should be administered as a 5% solution (50 g/l) or the bicarbonate can be dissolved in lactated Ringer's solution.

Antibiotics are of questionable value. They do not eliminate the organism from the gastrointestinal tract and may contribute to the carrier state. It has been claimed that prompt treatment of febrile, neutropenic horses with high therapeutic levels of suitable antibiotics may prevent them from developing diarrhoea. Suggested antibiotics include trimethoprim/sulphadoxine at 15 mg active ingredient/kg b.i.d. i.v., and some of the modern broad-spectrum semi-synthetic penicillins.

N.B. Parenteral tetracyclines should be avoided as they are excreted in the bile and may alter the gut flora, as would antibiotics given orally.

Codeine phosphate (0.2–2 g/kg) may slow down colon.

The use of non-steroidal anti-inflammatory drugs, e.g. phenylbutazone, has been suggested to reduce the fever, thereby indirectly improving the appetite. They may reduce prostaglandin synthesis, thus avoiding the active secretion of sodium and chloride into the intestine.

Control and public health considerations
Isolate all diarrhoeal cases until proven not to be shedding *Salmonella* organisms
Prevent dissemination of organisms from infected animal(s)

Clean and disinfect the box(es) after careful disposal of bedding and faeces
following death/recovery of the affected animal

Advise owner and attendants on hygiene rules when handling horses with
diarrhoea

Although the Zoonoses Order 1989 does not, at present, require mandatory
reporting of equine salmonellosis cases, it is important to carry out non-
statutory reporting of *Salmonella* isolates to improve the monitoring of
salmonellosis incidence at a national level

Equine intestinal clostridiosis

An acute diarrhoeal syndrome in which the intestinal flora has an
abnormally high number of *Clostridium perfringens*. Cases appear sporadically, apparently precipitated by stress, antibiotic therapy or diet.

In the adult horse, it has been associated with *C. perfringens* A and in foals
(where occasional outbreaks have been reported in 1–2-day-old foals), *C.
perfringens* B and C.

Clinical signs
Fever 39–40°C (102–104°F)

Acute depression and anorexia

Discoloured mucous membranes

Elevated pulse (75–140/min) and respiratory rate

Rapid dehydration

Mild abdominal pain

Peracute form – found dead with no evidence of diarrhoea

Acute form – sudden onset of severe clinical signs; explosive, watery diarrhoea

Mild form – acute onset of mild clinical signs, in particular anorexia,
depression and soft faeces

Diagnosis
Clinical signs supported by the presence of abnormally high counts of *C.
perfringens*, $>10^4$ colony-forming units per g faeces (<10 normal), with
the absence of *Salmonella* sp. in the faeces

Diagnostic aids
Haematology – early leucopenia (total WBC to 2500/ml), leucocytosis
follows (up to 25 000 WBC/ml), and elevation of packed cell volume
(PCV) (dehydration)

Blood chemistry – reflects damage to the parenchymatous organs, in particular the liver, and severe dehydration, e.g. increased total protein and
blood urea nitrogen

Treatment
Fluid therapy i.v. essential in the early stages
Antibiotics are justified as it is impossible to have a definite diagnosis in the
   early stages
Sour milk by stomach tube thought to contain a substance which selectively
   inhibits clostridial growth
A large dose of corticosteroid may increase the possibility of survival
Lamb dysentery serum prophylactically for foals at risk

Prognosis
Generally poor:
   peracute form usually found dead
   acute form die within 24–48 hours
   mild form tend to have a protracted course
   Complete recovery is possible with prompt treatment. There may be a
marked improvement in cases likely to survive after 1–2 days treatment but
relapses may occur.

Colitis X

An acute, often fatal, disease of the adult horse. Cases occur sporadically
and appear to be precipitated by stress or broad-spectrum antibiotic
therapy.

Clinical signs
Sudden onset depression
Discoloured ('dirty') mucous membranes
Elevated pulse rate (about 100/min)
Early fever of 39.5°C (103°F) soon falls to subnormal
Weakness, collapse, abdominal pain and death follow
Normal faeces if death within 3–4 hours with dehydration and profuse
   diarrhoea if the horse survives longer

Diagnosis
Following elimination of salmonellosis and intestinal clostridiosis a diagnosis of colitis X is usually made in cases of acute colitis in the horse.

Diagnostic aids
Haematology:
   there may be a leucopenia
   PCV may be as high as 70%
Blood chemistry: similar to intestinal clostridiosis

Differential diagnosis
Salmonellosis
Intestinal clostridiosis
Poisons (uncommon), e.g. arsenic, organophosphorus, rhododendron

Treatment
As for intestinal clostridiosis.

Prognosis
Many die within 24 hours. Horses which survive the first 24–48 hours tend to have a prolonged course with a generally unsatisfactory outcome.

Antibiotic-associated diarrhoea

The use of broad spectrum antibiotic therapy has been reported as a cause of diarrhoea in the horse, with tetracyclines specifically implicated when high doses have been used (approx. 30 mg/kg compared with the normal dose of 2–4 mg/kg).

Lincomycin, not recommended for use in the horse – when fed accidentally to horses (at 0.5 mg/kg) has been associated with diarrhoea.

Cases appear after the third day of treatment and are related to a prior 'stress', possibly the infection that antibiotics are being used to treat.

Clinical signs
Diarrhoea, possibly with blood present, preceded by depression, anorexia
    and mild abdominal pain
Severe dehydration

Treatment
General supportive therapy, with poor results in most cases

Prognosis
Mortality rate is high
Most cases die within 24 hours if the dehydration is not corrected

Anterior enteritis (duodenitis, proximal jejunitis)
Clinical signs
Acute onset colic
Rapid development of dehydration
Depression
Large volumes of fluid produced on nasogastric intubation, with relief of pain
May be distended small intestine palpable on rectal examination

Diagnosis

May be difficult to differentiate from small intestinal obstruction. Clearest indicator is the obvious pain relief following each removal of fluid by nasogastric intubation, followed by further signs of discomfort if stomach allowed to distend. Increased peritoneal fluid protein concentration also present.

Treatment

Usually medical but surgical intervention (duodenocaecostomy, jejuno-caecostomy and gastric decompression) may be tried in conjunction with medical management
Repeated nasogastric drainage
Intravenous electrolytes
Analgesia: flunixin only when satisfied with diagnosis
Antibacterials:
    penicillin
    metronidazole

Prognosis

Method of treatment, medical versus medical plus surgical intervention, does not appear to affect prognosis. Euthanasia should be considered if no apparent signs of improvement after several days of therapy. Reports suggest that horses which do not survive have a higher concentration of protein in the abdominal fluid and an increased anion gap.

Gastric ulceration

Thought to be frequently asymptomatic and possibly related to diet.

Clinical signs

Weight loss
Anaemia possible and hypoalbuminaemia if chronic blood loss
Mild colic/sweating especially after feeding

Treatment

Reduce concentrates until signs disappear
Most horses will get better
Ranitidine at 6.6 mg/kg t.i.d. orally for 14–21 days may help

Parasitic diarrhoea

See also Chapter 6.

Mixed strongyle infections

Larval cyathostomiasis is one of the commonest causes of chronic diarrhoea
Common in horses under five years of age in the winter/spring months.

Clinical signs

Diarrhoea – acute or chronic
Rapid or gradual weight loss
Numerous worms may be found in faeces on the disposable glove after rectal
    examination
In advanced cases:
    emaciation
    limb oedema
    elevated pulse and respiratory rates

Diagnosis

From history of grazing management and anthelmintic treatment, age of
horse and season, with clinical signs.

Diagnostic aids

Haematology: leucocytosis common and reflects severity
                eosinophilia uncommon
Blood chemistry – hypoalbuminaemia also reflects severity
                raised β-globulin (early *S. vulgaris* migration); if >25% of
                total protein, probably significant
Faecal examination – frequently negative (prepatent infection or recent
    worming). May give some indication of 'general state'

Treatment

Anthelmintics at larvicidal doses, e.g. fenbendazole at 60 mg/kg on one
    occasion or 5.5 mg/kg daily for five consecutive days, or ivermectin oral
    paste.
Supportive therapy – parenteral fluid as necessary, bandage tail, wash then
    smear perineum with vaseline.

Prognosis

Failure to respond may be due to permanent mucosal damage. If there
is to be a response, it is noticed 3–4 days after larvicidal anthelmintic therapy, but it may be 3–4 weeks before the horse passes completely normal
faeces.

    Salmonella organisms may be shed in the faeces in the early stages. It is of
little significance and ceases following anthelmintic treatment. As the
affected horse becomes more debilitated, an acute salmonellosis may
develop.

Coccidiosis – *Eimeria leuckarti*
Infection is most common in horses under one year of age, but clinical cases are rare despite *Eimeria leuckarti* being present in the small intestine.

Clinical signs
Diarrhoea of several days duration
Acute intestinal haemorrhage

Diagnosis
Eliminate the more common causes of diarrhoea as the isolation of the parasite does not in itself confirm the diagnosis.

Aid to diagnosis
Faecal examination – use sedimentation techniques or solutions of higher specific gravity if flotation techniques are used as the oöcysts are heavy.

Treatment
Coccidiosis can be a self-limiting disease and clinical signs subside spontaneously when the multiplication stage is passed. Sulphadimidine may assist in the treatment of clinical cases but there is insufficient information available to make reliable recommendations.

Equine intestinal trichomoniasis
Although it occurs in horses of all ages, it appears that colts of 2–3 years of age are most readily affected. Suckling foals appear to be resistant.

Clinical signs
Sudden onset, severe, greenish, watery diarrhoea
Fever of 40–42°C (103–108°F)
Depression, poor appetite
Rapid dehydration
Mild cases also found when soft (cow dung) faeces are passed

Diagnosis
A diagnosis can be made by microscopic examination of freshly collected faecal material for the presence of the organism.

Treatment
Trichomonicide – the specific trichomonicide, iodochlorhydroxyquin, is not available in the UK, but the use of a related compound, chlorhydroxyquinoline (Quixalud, Squibb), has been described
Reduce intestinal motility – atropine (50–100 mg/450 kg), diphenoxylate hydrochloride (Lomotil, Searle) at 400–700 mg/kg

Supportive therapy

Re-establish a normal intestinal flora – e.g. mix faeces from a clinically normal horse with water, strain the mixture and administer the extract by stomach tube

Prognosis

Some cases may die within 24 hours

If death does not occur, the disease may become chronic when the appetite improves but the diarrhoea persists along with progressive dehydration and emaciation

In mild cases there is a recovery in 3–4 weeks with supportive therapy

It may take 3–6 months for complete normality to be restored, with relapses common when horses come off treatment. The whole treatment procedure must then be started again

Other causes of diarrhoea

In cases of diarrhoea the cause may never be established. Many cases of diarrhoea are due to improper feeding and bad management. Regular feeding of good hay and good quality concentrates, which have been stored correctly, is essential if the non-specific diarrhoeas are to be avoided.

In cases of diarrhoea of apparently unknown aetiology check for the following:
- Access to or contamination of the foodstuffs by poisons, e.g. arsenic
- The presence of poisonous plants in the pasture or hay
- Inadvertent or unknowing addition of therapeutic agent(s) to food or the feeding of foodstuffs intended for another species
- The possible contamination by, or development (by incorrect storage) of significant levels of, for example, moulds or mycotoxins

If one is still unable to make a diagnosis, it is advisable to administer anthelmintic in a larvicidal dose on the first or second visit

Malabsorption syndromes

Malabsorption, protein-losing enteropathy and chronic diarrhoea are not synonymous, but some conditions involve all three, with most cases multifactorial in origin. Attempts must be made to identify the region of gut involved.

Granulomatous bowel disease

Similar to Crohn's disease in humans, when a diffuse mononuclear infiltration of the small intestine (ileum in particular) leads to malabsorption and albumin loss.

Clinical signs
Continued weight loss over a period of months
Normal appetite
Diarrhoea in 50% of cases
Subcutaneous oedema later

Diagnosis
On clinical signs supported by laboratory findings.

Diagnostic aids
Blood chemistry:
  hypoalbuminaemia
  flat oral glucose tolerance test
Histopathology:
  on intestinal biopsy (gut wall macroscopically has a thickened, corru-
  gated appearance, with raised, pinkish, plaque-like lesions on the serosa)

Treatment
None, other than trying corticosteroids.

Prognosis
Poor.

Inadequate absorptive surface
Following intestinal resection, > 50% of small intestine.

Idiopathic villous atrophy
Has occurred in young thoroughbreds.

Clinical signs
Persistent weight loss
May have increased appetite
May have diarrhoea

Diagnosis
From history, clinical signs, elimination of other causes of weight loss. The
use of the glucose and D-xylose absorption tests may confirm that malabsorption is present.

Treatment
None known to be effective.

Intestinal tuberculosis
Infection is invariably by the oral route with granulomatous lesions in the intestinal mucosa, mesenteric lymph nodes and spleen.

Clinical signs
Chronic weight loss
Enlarged mesenteric lymph nodes on rectal examination
Peritoneal effusion
Diarrhoea is uncommon

Diagnosis
It is difficult to differentiate intestinal tuberculosis from neoplastic changes
without laboratory assistance, unless acid-fast organism found on smear
or biopsy
Intradermal tests are unreliable in the horse

Diagnostic aids
Histopathology – examination of a biopsy
Faecal examination:
smears – stain and look for acid-fast bacilli
culture – may take too long

Treatment
On confirmation of the diagnosis, destroy affected animals.
Care: *Zoonosis*

Protein-losing enteropathy
Usually present in inflammatory or infiltrative disorders and important in terms of overall effect. Some may be immune mediated, others affected by dietary constituents, infectious agents and internal parasites.

Investigation of malabsorption syndromes

History
Age
Management changes
Feed and worming regimes
Duration and rapidity of progression
Presence of diarrhoea or colic

Examination
Check for weight loss, muscle wasting
Presence of oedema
Demeanour

Aids to diagnosis
Care – easy to run up expensive clinical pathology bills in cases with poor or
    hopeless prognosis
Routine haematology
Total protein (with electrophoresis) and albumin
Urea and creatinine
AST
GGT
Fibrinogen

Subsequently
Glucose absorption
Xylose absorption
Lactose tolerance (foals)
Liver function tests $\pm$ biopsy
Laparotomy and gut biopsies

Alimentary tract neoplasia

Three of the most commonly encountered types follow.

Oesophageal squamous cell carcinoma
Presents with a history of recurrent oesophageal obstruction. Diagnosis is by
fibreoptoscopic examination of the oesophagus, contrast radiography and/or
finding neoplastic squamous cells in the pleural fluid.

Gastric squamous cell carcinoma
The commonest type of gastric tumour. The clinical signs include chronic
weight loss, poor appetite, anaemia, and on occasions recurrent oesophageal
obstruction. Diagnosis is from exploratory laparotomy, although an
abnormal mass may be felt on rectal examination in some cases.

Alimentary lymphosarcoma
The multicentric, alimentary, cutaneous and thymic forms occur in the
horse. Alimentary tract involvement may be diffuse or localized. Clinical
signs include weight loss, diarrhoea, subcutaneous oedema and enlarged
mesenteric lymph nodes or spleen on rectal examination.

Other than exploratory laparotomy and biopsy, diagnosis can be assisted
by the presence of a leucocytosis, predominantly lymphocytes (total WBC
>16 000ml) or finding a lymphocytosis and atypical cells on abdominal
paracentesis.

A localized alimentary lymphosarcoma can occur and causes intestinal
obstruction due to the local growth of the tumour.

Oesophageal obstruction

Usually as a sequel to the rapid ingestion of food. The common foods implicated include sugar beet pulp (inadequately soaked) and nuts, pelleted foods, windfall apples, etc.

Clinical signs
Horse is frequently distressed with saliva discharging, possibly with food, from the nostrils
Drooling saliva
Coughing
Head and neck arched with pain as swallowing attempts are made
Respiratory signs, if there is an aspiration pneumonia, appear after 12–24 hours

Diagnosis
Clinical signs are usually diagnostic
Passage of a stomach tube may confirm the presence of an obstruction

Aids to diagnosis
Oesophageal endoscopy
Contrast media radiography

Treatment
In the first instance the horse will probably require sedation to allow a proper examination. This sedation can assist in the passage of the stomach tube to confirm the diagnosis
Analgesics – should have antispasmolytic activity
Atropine – helps to reduce salivation
Lubricant – a small amount of liquid paraffin (100 ml)
Water – to try to soften material (should only be used with general anaesthesia and intubation with a cuffed endotracheal tube if attempts are made to flush out the material)
Antibiotics – if fever or abnormal lung sounds are present
Surgery – if medical treatment fails or is considered unsuitable.
This should be decided upon early, as a persistent obstruction causes mucosal necrosis and inflammation of the oseophageal wall within 48 hours

Prognosis
Good for removal of the obstruction by medical treatments
Failure or recurrent obstructions usually result from diverticulum formation or oesophageal neoplasia

Colic

Colic is the name for abdominal pain. As far as the owners are concerned it refers to the behavioural manifestations of this pain. It is not a diagnosis or specific disease.

Pain may arise from distension, spasm or ischaemia of the gastro-intestinal tract. It may arise from tension on, or stretching of, the mesentery and from peritonitis. Always treat calmly, quickly and compassionately.

Colic cases are potential emergencies and should be treated as such. Most respond well to medical treatment, but it is essential that the clinician is able to differentiate the more serious cases, as a surgical colic has a greatly reduced prognosis more than eight hours after the onset of clinical signs.

Colic cases require regular reassessment by the clinician.

If a colic is to be referred, ensure the owners have correct directions and the referral centre has an accurate arrival time (but assessed once horse loaded). Consider welfare implications of transport (Transit of Animals Regulations apply). Give analgesia if necessary, best after discussion with referral centre. Decompress stomach and, if necessary, travel with tube *in situ*. Send written details of clinical findings, and *all* medication given and timings, with relevant samples of blood or peritoneal fluid.

History
This is important and may be taken while observing the horse
Duration of clinical signs
Nature of pain and frequency of episodes if intermittent
Appetite
Faeces – nature, quantity and when last passed
Urine – when last seen passing urine, nature, volume, and any difficulty
State of nutrition and feeding regime
Parasite control product used, dose, when last given and frequency of normal wormings
Previous medical history
Work prior to colic

Common signs seen in colic
Restlessness
Sweating
Pawing the ground
Kicking or looking at the abdomen
Rolling, lying on the ground or getting up and down
Anorexia
Constipation or diarrhoea

Straddled position with straining

Depression with severe shock in those terminally ill, with few signs of colic

Clinical examination

If horse is in great distress, give analgesic. Before entering box, be aware of safety of personnel and always exercise great care

The clinical examination should enable the cause to be classified, with specific emphasis on differentiation of surgical from medical cases at an early stage

Temperature

Pulse and respiratory rate

Degree of pain

Sweating – type

Mucous membrane colour and capillary refill time

Abdominal auscultation which should be used to monitor progress. Gut sounds and propulsive activity are not synonymous. Complete silence indicates severe lesion

Percussion and assess presence of distension, tucked-up/board-like appearance

Rectal examination, unless character of horse does not permit it to be done safely

Abdominal paracentesis

Foals – transabdominal palpation

Nasogastric intubation: quantities of fluid in grass disease, gastric emptying impairment, small intestinal blockage and gastroduodenitis. If blood present, may be ulceration, neoplasia or strangulating obstruction

Aids to diagnosis

Haematology

Packed cell volume estimation is easily carried out in the field, with a battery-operated portable haematocrit. A rise in PCV to 50–70% indicates immediate fluid therapy, and, if at 70%, suggests a serious colic which is producing hypovolaemic shock when euthanasia should be considered

Total leucocyte count and differential

Blood chemistry

Total serum protein, glucose and lactate are measures of circulatory failure

Other than leucocyte count the above parameters rise in serious colic

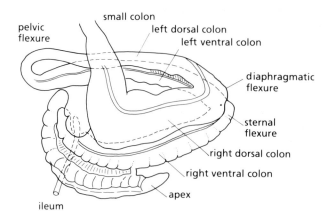

Fig. 2.2 Diagram of the caecum and large colon.

Rectal examination

Most commonly no abnormality is detected

Firm, dry faeces in the rectum or large colon – possible impaction – ensure pelvic flexure and caecum, the most common sites, are identified and palpated (see Fig. 2.2)

Distension of viscera by gas or gas and fluid – check for tight bands, in particular on small colon and mesentery

Palpable mass:

abscess

tumour, e.g. lipoma

pregnancy

aneurism

Any displacement of abdominal viscera

Smoothness of peritoneum

Paracentesis abdominis

Spasmodic colic – normal

Tympanitic – normal

Impaction (primary) – normal

Ischaemic lesions – amber to red to dark red colour, elevated protein and red blood cells (RBC) present

Intestinal rupture – dark yellow/brown colour, very high WBC count, food or faecal material may be present (repeat paracentesis at other site in case needle was in gut lumen)

A specific indication of intestinal insult is obtained when there is a rapid (in less than two hours) rise in level of the intestinal isoenzyme of alkaline phosphatase

Bacteria on smear generally from bowel rupture unless within leucocytes, which suggests bowel necrosis

Classification of colic

Spasmodic
Probably the most common form encountered
It is usually transient, relapsing and self-limiting
Most cases respond to antispasmolytic drugs

Clinical signs
Sudden onset
Periods when pain is present with the horse apparently normal or near normal in between. May be transient or last several hours
Pulse rate up to 70/min with respiratory rate elevated during bouts of pain
Gut sounds present which may be more pronounced
On rectal examination and stomach tubing no abnormal findings

Diagnosis
On clinical signs and response to treatment.

Treatment
Analgesic and antispasmolytic drugs – see Chapter 14.

Tympanitic
A common type where fermentation leads to production of gas which distends the stomach or intestines; found most commonly in horses fed a highly fermentative diet, such as unsuitable food, e.g. grass cuttings, fallen apples or sudden changes in concentrate diet. It may be from overproduction of, or failure to void, the gas. It is usually self-limiting.

Clinical signs
Continuous pain
Pulse rate up to 80/min and rising in severe cases
Gut sounds reduced
Gastric distension may be present
Stomach tubing gives gas and fluid reflux in gastric tympany
Rectal examination:
    intestinal – distended portions palpable
    spleen may be displaced caudally

Diagnosis
From clinical signs with history of feeding fermentative foods

Any lack of response to treatment, rapid recurrence or increase in signs
indicates a possible 'surgical colic'

Treatment
Analgesics – may be necessary before a complete examination is achieved

If overeating suspected, flunixin i.v. (or other non-steroid anti-inflammatory
drug (NSAID)) to protect against the effect of endotoxaemia

Stomach tube cases of gastric tympany

Gut-active antibiotics orally, linseed oil or turpentine oil may combat the
fermentation

Exploratory laparotomy if cases of intestinal tympany do not respond to
analgesics and antifermentative agents, or the pulse rate exceeds 80/min
with an increasing PCV

Prognosis
Good in most cases but fermentation may give endotoxaemia and laminitis.

Obstructive (ileus)
Mechanical – from lumen obstruction, extralumenal compression or
topographical alterations. Any compression may produce ischaemic
damage

Paralytic – from decreased intestinal motility

Small intestinal obstruction

Mechanical
Herniation
Intussusception
Volvulus
Pedunculate lipomas
Adhesions

Impactions
Ileocaecal valve
Ascarids

Large intestinal obstruction

Mechanical
Torsion of large colon or caecum (or partial torsion)
Volvulus of small colon

Impactions (very common)
Caecal

Small colon
Large colon (most frequent)

The 'obstruction' may be due to failure of peristalsis of ischaemic or neurogenic origin:

Ischaemic bowel disease
Recent research indicates that the obstruction to blood flow is mediated at the mural vessel level, when either a local intravascular coagulation or vasoconstriction takes place. Primarily affects small intestine and caecum (colon to a lesser extent).

Neurogenic
Characterized by a neurogenic paralytic ileus affecting any or all intestinal segments between pharynx and anus. (See Grass sickness, p. 54).

The severity and rate of progression of clinical signs in obstructive colics depend upon
1 Degree of obstruction.
2 Rapidity of visceral distension.
3 Degree of vascular compromise.
4 Surface area involved through which bacteria and toxins can escape.
   Impactions follow abrupt changes in diet, reduced water consumption, dental problems and feeding at irregular intervals. A reduction in volume and type of faeces may have been noticed before colic.

Large intestinal impactions

Clinical signs
Insidious in onset over a number of days when dry, hard faeces are passed
   before the animal is obviously abnormal
Anorexia
Dull, continuous pain – sternal and diaphragmatic flexures more painful
Pulse rate of 40–50/min
Reduced gut sounds
Dry, hard faeces in rectum, pelvic flexure or caecum

Diagnosis
From the suggestive clinical signs confirmed on rectal examination by palpation of the impaction. In small ponies rectal examination may be impossible and initial treatment started on the provisional diagnosis and response to treatment allows a retrospective diagnosis to be made.

Treatment

Laxatives – liquid paraffin (1 litre/90 kg) by stomach tube is an excellent lubricant but does not penetrate the faeces as well as surfactant agents. Repeated administration over several days is necessary.

Purgatives – most respond to the liquid paraffin but it may be necessary to promote peristalsis, but only if the impaction is soft, if there is no necrosis of the intestinal wall and the lumen is patent. 250 g $MgSO_4$ in 3–4 litres of water following previous use of liquid paraffin.

Analgesics – morphine derivatives will cause powerful muscular contractions in the small intestine.

Enema – most beneficial in meconium retention in the foal.

Surgical intervention – indicated in non-responsive cases. Caecal impaction very difficult to clear by medical treatment.

Small intestinal impactions

Clinical signs
Sudden onset with rapid progression to:
- Severe continuous abdominal pain
- Pulse rate 70–80/min and rising
- Gut sounds almost totally absent after the first 1–2 hours
- Regurgitation of stomach contents through stomach tube or nose
- Distended bowel *may not* be palpated on rectal examination

Diagnosis
From the clinical signs.

Treatment
Prompt surgical intervention.

Enteritis induced
Any acute or peracute disease of the bowel will produce abdominal pain. The high fever and profound neutropenia are useful diagnostic aids. In these cases the most important microbial cause is salmonellosis, which should be remembered if the horse is to be taken to a veterinary centre for examination and treatment.

Endotoxaemia and intestinal ischaemia
Compromise of the intestinal wall allows movement of bacterial endotoxin across the wall and into the systemic circulation.

Clinical signs
Early – pyrexia, bright pink mucous membranes, decreased CRT, tachycardia

Later – normal or decreased temperature, muddy to cyanotic mucous
   membranes. Sweating, colic and dyspnoea
Haemoconcentration and disseminated intravascular coagulation (DIC)
develop
WBC decrease early with leucocytosis if horse survives
   Many effects are mediated by prostaglandin/thromboxane pathways.
Flunixin meglumine is best at preventing or reducing the early effects of
endotoxaemia – hypoxaemia, pulmonary hypertension, colic and intestinal
fluid loss.

Treatment

Fluids – balanced electrolyte unless laboratory facilities available to indicate
   more specific requirements
Flunixin better than prednisolone, dexamethasone or phenylbutazone
Antibiotics – broad spectrum
DMSO for anti-inflammatory, analgesic, diuretic actions
Heparin – 40 iu/kg t.i.d., s.c. or i.v. to decrease the PCV or 100 iu/kg t.i.d.
   i.v. for anticoagulant effect

Peritonitis

Peritonitis is a complication of surgical colic but may occur spontaneously. Gastrointestinal rupture, rectal tears and effusions from neoplastic lesions may produce peritonitis associated with signs of acute
abdominal crisis.
   The signs are of generalized abdominal pain with increased heart rate,
varying degree of dehydration and circulatory dysfunction.

Peritoneal fluid

Common findings are elevated nucleated cell count to $< 10^{10}$/l with haematological abnormalities and elevated plasma fibrinogen. Culture fluid
both aerobically and anaerobically. Protein level gives a quick assessment.

Treatment

Immediate treatment with broad spectrum antibiotics, e.g. penicillin and
streptomycin; penicillin, trimethoprim/sulphonamide; amoxycillin, tri-
methoprim/sulphonamide combinations. Continue until clinical response
and for at least seven days.
   Non-steroidal anti-inflammatory agents – use flunixin *only* when certain
it is not a surgical colic.
Intravenous fluid therapy as necessary.

Surgical or possible surgical cases

Do revisit and reassess colic cases, unless the owner telephones to say the
horse is fully recovered, rather than saying 'phone me if it's not better'.

Do refer them early – even if the case turns out only to require medical
treatment. Time is of the essence if the surgeon is to have an opportunity
to carry out successful surgery. The prognosis for a surgical colic is
greatly reduced if presented more than eight hours after the onset of
clinical signs.

Do not give acetylpromazine if anaesthesia and surgery might follow, as the
hypotensive action provides a serious complication. If it is necessary to
relieve distress, even to make examination more simple, xylazine can be
used although its potent analgesic effects only last for 30–60 minutes.
Detomidine, although a potent analgesic, should not be used as it will
mask the clinical signs over too long a period of time for the clinician to
be aware of any deterioration in the horse's condition.

Grass sickness

An equine dysautonomia, grass sickness affects all equine species and occurs
throughout the UK with a similar condition reported in Germany, Sweden
and Australia. Although there is a seasonal incidence, cases do occur all
year. The incidence is usually one animal but multiple incidence within a
group has been reported, usually in animals at grass.

Three forms of the disease are recognized as follows:

Peracute/acute

Sudden onset with rapidly progressing symptoms of depression, anorexia,
abdominal pain, sweating, fine muscle tremors, elevated pulse rate (to 100/
min), inability to swallow, absent or very reduced gut sounds and progressive dehydration. A green nasal discharge is commonly seen. Gastric
dilation present and gastric rupture is possible.

Animals seldom survive more than 2–3 days, with an occasional one
dying within 24 hours of the onset of clinical signs. If a diagnosis of peracute
or acute grass sickness is made, euthanasia should be advised.

N.B. With degree of gastric distension likely, decompress stomach
frequently. If sending to referral centre, do so with nasogastric tube *in situ*.

Subacute

Onset is less sudden with the signs taking a few days to develop. The clinical
signs are less severe than in the acute and the characteristic green nasal
discharge is not seen in many of the cases.

The course of the disease is more protracted. Animals may last up to 1–2 weeks with the mortality rate close to 100%. The survivors may become chronic cases.

Chronic

Progressive weight loss – leads to emaciation and weakness
Difficulty in eating and drinking
Small quantities of faeces, if any, passed

The majority progress to such thinness and weakness that euthanasia is carried out, or the animal dies, but occasional recoveries are thought to occur.

Diagnosis

Clinical signs difficult to differentiate from other causes of colic
Barium studies show defective oesophageal motility (barium pooling)

Grass sickness cases have been found to have higher specific gravity and protein content than medical colic cases although appearance of fluid is similar. Surgical cases have bloodstained fluid with a higher alkaline phosphatase activity.

Confirmation of the disease is at post-mortem examination when degenerative change is found in the coeliaco-mesenteric and thoracic sympathetic ganglia.

Although it can be very difficult to make a definite diagnosis, do not allow cases of grass sickness to drag on. Avoid high risk premises especially in April, May and June, if possible.

Abdominal abscess

See Chapter 1.

3 / Liver disease

Clinical signs of liver dysfunction are due to the inability of the affected organ to fulfil its metabolic, synthetic and excretory functions. The liver has a reserve capacity and an unusual ability to regenerate, allowing mild insults to be generally well tolerated. If this is exceeded by massive acute or persistent chronic damage the clinical signs of liver disease are shown.

Types of liver disease

Primary liver disease (see below)
Secondary liver disease – from endotoxins causing hepatic damage, e.g. in septicaemias and acute alimentary tract conditions

Primary liver disease
1 From damage to hepatocytes (acute or chronic).
2 Bile duct obstruction.
3 Hyperlipaemia.

Hepatocyte damage

Acute form
Acute hepatitis
    thought to be viral in origin
    leptospirosis
    may follow administration of homologous serum
Chemical toxicities – lead, arsenic, carbon tetrachloride

Chronic form
Ragwort poisoning – damage is chronic but clinical signs appear as acute encephalopathy
Tyzzer's disease – see Chapter 5

Clinical signs

Acute form
Sudden onset of clinical signs
Anorexia
Abdominal pain with markedly elevated pulse and respiratory rates
Icterus is a prominent, early sign in more than 80% of cases

Progressive central nervous system (CNS) signs may be seen with circling, head pressing, ataxia, mania and convulsions possible

Urine may be discoloured

Photosensitization may follow

Chronic form

More common form of the disease

CNS signs predominate

Head pressing

Depression

Abnormal gait and stance

Depraved appetite

These signs are progressive with the animal eventually unable to stand. In addition there may be:

Weight loss

Ventral oedema

Diarrhoea or soft faeces

Icterus

Photosensitization

May have sudden onset of signs as liver failure progresses

Diagnosis

From the history and clinical signs supported by diagnostic tests.

Differential diagnosis

Colic

Lead poisoning

Botulism

Tetanus

Rabies

CNS space-occupying lesion

Diagnostic aids

Haematology

    total white blood cells (WBC) increased with shift to left

    packed cell volume (PCV) increased in acute cases

    haemoglobinaemia in acute cases

Blood chemistry

Bilirubin – elevated in chronic and acute cases, both direct and indirect levels must be monitored

Liver enzymes – serve as a guide to continuous liver damage

    aspartate aminotransferase (AST) – not liver specific, elevated in acute damage

sorbitol dehydrogenase (SDH) – liver specific, elevated in acute damage
lactate dehydrogenase (LDH) – not liver specific, elevated in acute damage
gamma glutamyltransferase (GGT) – mainly elevated in chronic disease but also in acute hepatitis
Bromsulphalein (BSP) clearance – an excellent diagnostic aid in chronic and borderline cases but unreliable in markedly icteric animals
Blood urea nitrogen – useful in evaluating functional failure
Blood ammonia – not always elevated. If levels exceed 90 mmol/l CNS signs may be anticipated. Must be done very rapidly after sampling
Liver biopsy – see Chapter 15
Urine analysis – is useful with bilirubinuria indicating liver disease and haemoglobinuria indicating severe damage

Treatment
Therapy is mainly symptomatic and supportive to allow time for regeneration
Antibacterials – for primary and secondary bacterial infection and to limit urea splitting bacteria, e.g. oral neomycin 40–60/400 kg divided daily
Vitamin supplements – vitamin B complex, vitamin K and methionine e.g. 100–200 mg thiamine/24 hours
Blood glucose levels should be maintained with intravenous dextrose solution, or oral, 5 g/kg/24 hours
Sedation – to control CNS signs
Management changes:
    keep horse out of sunlight
    laxatives to limit ammonia production – liquid paraffin
    low protein diet with added glucose
    oral electrolytes during the recovery period

Prognosis
Very poor. Acute hepatitis: up to 90% die. If maniacal form presents, consider euthanasia early, N.B. owner and vet safety!

Ragwort poisoning
Although this presents as an acute encephalopathy it is usually a sequel to a chronic development. The horse is unaware of its surroundings, and shows head pressing, circling, weight loss, diarrhoea and subcutaneous oedema.

Prevention is important – pull and burn ragwort before seeding. Check the hay for the presence of the dried plant – *do not feed* hay which contains ragwort.

Bile duct obstruction

May be caused by liver fluke, space-occupying lesion(s) such as pancreatic tumours or cholelithiasis, or ascarid impaction.

Clinical signs are pain from stretching of visceral peritoneum presenting as colic. Those of obstructive jaundice and differentiation from other causes of jaundice can be assisted by laboratory tests:

Bilirubin – direct component mainly elevated

Enzyme estimation – staphylococcus aureus protease (SAP) elevated in obstructive jaundice

BSP clearance – unreliable in markedly icteric cases as a total bilirubin of greater than 100 mmol/l interferes with the test

Exploratory laparotomy may be indicated, when cholelithiasis can possibly be broken down or removed.

Hyperlipaemia

Occurs in ponies, often if pregnant and underfed or inappetant and unable to utilize the triglyceride resulting in fatty degeneration of the liver and kidney. Fat mobilization is increased when a horse or pony is deprived of food which results in a high level of plasma triglyceride. These factors, with stress and lactation, are associated with peripheral resistance to the action of insulin, which in man results in poor regulation of adipose lipolysis, increased plasma free fatty acid (FFA) concentration and hypertriglyceridaemia. A case has been seen where this condition was produced by the over zealous feeding of cod liver oil to a two-year-old Shire show horse.

Clinical signs are non-specific but lethargy, inappetance, oedema and diarrhoea are seen. Underlying or concurrent disease may be present. A typical opaque white (milky) or yellow fatty plasma and elevated total blood lipid and triglyceride levels are found. Evidence of hepatopathy may also be found with a fatty liver on biopsy.

Treatment is to correct the predisposing cause and improve the food intake with general supportive therapy. The cause of any anorexia must be treated and food intake increased by offering grass or even feeding a slurry or feed cubes by stomach tube.

Heparin up to 250 iu/kg bid. (5000 iu/day for a Shetland) has been successful.

Insulin, for a 200 kg pony, 30 iu protamine zinc insulin i/m b.i.d. + 100 g glucose orally on every second day with 15 iu protamine zinc insulin i.m. + galactose orally b.i.d. on the alternate days. Feeding of a controlled intake ration is beneficial to improved insulin sensitivity, even in the absence of exercise, which is also beneficial.

Prognosis

Prognosis must be poor with over 50% mortality probable.

Despite the increased plasma triglyceride concentrations of up to 80-fold present, some workers consider the outcome unrelated to the degree of hypertriglyceridaemia.

Any pony which is dull and inappetant should be tested for hyperlipaemia to ensure early correction of any underlying disease and correction of energy balance.

4 / Urinary tract disease

Urinary tract disorders are less frequently recognized as clinical entities in the horse than in other species, despite pathological changes being not uncommon findings at routine post-mortem examination.

The principal signs of urinary tract disease include abnormal volumes of urine passed with or without changes in the constituents of the urine, abnormal frequency, and may include dysuria and pain on micturition.

Horse urine is normally more or less opaque, becoming more turbid towards the end of micturition. Clear urine is generally considered abnormal in the horse.

History
Important points include:
- Daily water intake
- Daily urine output, frequency and consistency
- Any weight loss, depression or anorexia

Clinical examination
Always include rectal examination – the left kidney (usually the only one that can be palpated this way), ureters and bladder. Particular attention should be given to any part of the urinary tract from which pain is elicited during this examination.

Aids to diagnosis
Laboratory evaluations (see Chapter 16) are necessary to establish the presence and severity of urinary tract disease:
Haematology
Biochemistry
Urine analysis
Sodium suphanilate clearance
Water deprivation test
Renal biopsy

Treatment
Preferable to use a drug which is actively excreted by the kidney, e.g. trimethoprim, sulphonamides, penicillin
Encourage water intake

Renal disease

Usually not detected in the early stages, with the history and clinical examination infrequently providing clear evidence of renal disease. Examination of a horse for another complaint may reveal abnormal results indicative of renal disease.

Pyelonephritis

May occur as an ascending infection or as a sequel to a septicaemia.

Clinical signs
Fever, but may not be present in advanced cases
Pus and blood in the urine
Abdominal pain
Renal enlargement and pain on palpation

Diagnosis
The presence of pus and blood in the urine is suggestive but must be
    differentiated from cystitis
Blood urea and creatinine levels may be elevated

Treatment
Antibacterial therapy – isolate the bacteria and determine their sensitivity to antibiotics and sulphonamides. Treatment is required for 7–10 days and repeated bacteriological examination of the urine is required to ensure that the infection has been completely controlled.

Nephrosis

1   Tubular nephrosis – may be associated with haemoglobinuria, myoglobinuria, chemical poisonings and some toxic heavy metals (e.g. mercury). Clinical signs are rarely seen but tubular degeneration has been reported as a post-mortem finding.
2   Glomerular nephrosis – possibly related to deposition of immune complexes and may follow severe infections. Reported cases have shown renal failure and died.
3   Hydronephrosis – cystic enlargement of a kidney, either congenital or as a result of ureter obstruction.
    Clinical signs are usually absent if the condition is unilateral, although a grossly distended kidney may be detected on rectal examination. With bilateral involvement there is uraemia and grossly distended kidneys detectable on rectal examination. Establishing the blood creatinine level and

use of the sodium sulphanilate clearance test will assist in diagnosing renal disease and may help in giving a more definitive prognosis.

Nephritis

A rare condition in the horse other than *Actinobacillus* infection in newborn foals.

1 Embolic suppurative nephritis – focal lesions occur in the kidneys following a bacteraemia, such as *Streptococcus equi* infection or other chronic streptococcal infections.

2 Interstitial nephritis – has been described in horses with a history of weight loss over a period of six months despite symptomatic treatment. Analysis of urine samples showed a high level of protein and a low-normal specific gravity.

3 Renal calculi – if present they do not appear to show symptoms (see below).

Cystitis

Inflammation of the bladder caused by bacteria, usually accompanied by urethritis.

Clinical signs
Frequent urination – small volumes of urine on each occasion
Pain on passing urine and may continue to stand and strain as if passing urine for some time afterwards
Blood, inflammatory cells and bacteria present in urine
Fever
Inappetance

Diagnosis
The frequent passing of small volumes of urine containing the products of inflammation
Pain with/without thickened bladder on rectal examination
Urinalysis when cells, casts and bacteria likely to be present

Differential diagnosis
Pyelonephritis – very difficult in many cases. In chronic and severe cases of cystitis some change may be detectable in the bladder wall on rectal examination. Provided the bacteria are identified and antibiotic sensitivity established, the treatment will be correct even if a wrong decision is made
Urolithiasis – calculi in the bladder will probably be palpable on rectal examination

Treatment

Antibacterial therapy – antibiotic sensitivity of bacteria isolated from the
  urine should be established. The treatment is required for 7–10 days and
  further samples of urine must be submitted for bacteriological examination to ensure that complete removal of infection has been achieved
  before therapy ceases

Water – free access to water at all times is essential to ensure a free flow of
  urine

Alter urinary pH – the use of hexamine and mandelic acid has been suggested but these are at best bacteriostatic

Urolithiasis

Urinary calculi occur anywhere in the urinary tract.

Vesical calculi

The bladder is the most common site for urinary calculi in the horse.

Clinical signs

Abdominal pain – usually mild
May walk with a stilted gait
Blood or clots may be present in the urine
Cystitis may be present
Dysuria possible

Diagnosis

Rectal examination – with the bladder empty

Treatment

Surgical removal

Urethral calculi

Clinical signs

Restlessness
Frequent attempts to pass urine
Colic
Bladder distended
Blood and debris in urine

Diagnosis

The calculi may be detected on passing a catheter. Crystalluria will probably
be present

Treatment

Smooth muscle relaxants may allow expulsion of the calculi. In the male it may be necessary to perform a urethrotomy.

Psychological polydipsia with polyuria

Cases of horses with significantly increased daily water intake and an obvious increase in daily output have been reported. A water deprivation test can be carried out in these cases and if required subsequently the anti-diuretic hormone (ADH) deficiency test.

Boredom has been found to be a reason for the polydipsia which will cease when the horse is moved to a box in the busiest part of the yard or to another yard. Horses with this problem should not be allowed automatic water bowls as this may also be aetiologically significant.

Urinary incontinence

Rare in horses.

Commonest cause is with the presence of discrete cystic calculi or diseases resulting in paralysis of the bladder and urethral musculature, such as equine herpes virus, myeloencephalitis, cauda equina neuritis or damage to vertebrae.

Prognosis is poor, if not hopeless in the long term, other than when the primary problem is cystic calculi.

5 / Foal diseases

Definitions

Minimum limit for viability is 300 days post-conception

Premature foal – born at 300–325 days gestation, which if under-developed is unlikely to survive

Immature foal (dysmature) – born at 325–355 days gestation showing similar evidence of underdevelopment – low birth weight, soft, silky coat, domed head, flexor tendon laxity, weak and with more severely affected cases, central nervous system (CNS) depression

Perinatal period – that time immediately before, during and after parturition up to and including normal sucking behaviour

Neonatal period – that period from birth to 14 days

Parameters by which a newborn foal can be judged

Standing

A foal should stand within 1 hour of birth (foals have been seen to stand as early as 20 minutes). If the foal has not been standing by 2 hours it should be regarded as possibly abnormal.

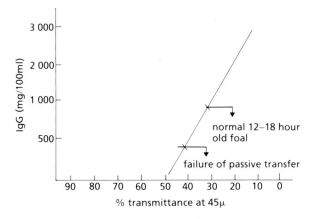

Fig. 5.1 Estimation of IgG levels by measurement of the transmittance of the serum with a spectrophotometer. If done at 12–18 hours of age there is time to administer colostrum orally to foals with low IgG levels.

Sucking

Thoroughbred foals have been seen to suck at between 35 and 420 minutes (mean of 111 minutes) and cross-bred foals at between 45 and 135 minutes (mean of 65 minutes). Foals that do not suck within 3 hours may be abnormal. Premature or weak foals may require colostrum by stomach tube.

Failure of immunity
Failure of passive transfer:
> 25% partial
> 10% total

1 Low immunoglobulin (Ig) colostral content (see Fig. 5.1)
2 Premature lactation
3 Premature parturition
4 Weak foal, mare's temperament, separation impeding access to colostrum
5 Malabsorption

Foals up to 12 hours of age
Oral colostrum – 500 ml followed by a further 500 ml in divided doses over the next 4 hours
Oral donor plasma – 1 litre by stomach tube over several feeds

Foals over 12 hours of age
Plasma i.v. at 20 ml/kg prophylactically or 30–40 ml/kg if infection suspected or present
> N.B. It is best to cross-match plasma with foal red blood cells (RBC). If facility not available, use plasma from gelding

Newborn foals tolerate bovine colostrum and can absorb bovine IgG. Despite a half-life of bovine IgG which is considerably shorter than the reported half-life for passively derived equine IgG in foals, it is an acceptable substitute source of immunoglobulins if equine colostrum is not available.

Meconium

Starts to be voided from 4 hours after birth with it being 'cleared' by 96 hours. In an occasional foal the signs associated with the passing of meconium may be seen at 1 hour post-partum. Colt foals are more commonly affected than filly foals, with an overall incidence of between 1% and 2%.

Rectal temperature

Immediately after birth it falls to 37°C, rising to 38°C (98.4°F rising to

100.5°F) by 1 hour post-partum. The rectal temperature can be measured every 6 hours to check for transitory rises.

Heart rate

At birth	60–80 beats/minute
1–12 hours	120–140 beats/minute
12 hours on	80–120 beats/minute

Heart murmur (ductus and foramen ovale) should disappear by 96 hours.

Respiratory rate

At birth	60–70 breaths/minute
1–12 hours	30–40 breaths/minute

Laboratory finding

Packed cell volume (PCV) – approximately 45 at birth decreasing to 40 at 48 hours

RBC count (total) – approximately $10 \times 10^{12}/l$ at birth decreasing to $8.5–9 \times 10^{12}/l$ after 36 hours

Haemoglobin – approximately 15 g/l at birth decreasing to 13 g/l at 48 hours

Leucocyte count (total) – $10 \times 10^9/l$ at 12 hours decreasing to $7–8 \times 10^9/l$ after 36 hours

Blood urea – less than 20 mg% (4 mmol/l)

Urine – proteinuria common in the first 36 hours

Assessment of immune status – zinc sulphate turbidity test

Abnormal findings

Tachycardia common in:
  septicaemia
  convulsions
  haemolytic disease
Tachypnoea after two hours:
  pulmonary problem – atelectasis
  pneumonia
  metabolic acidosis
Elevated rectal temperature – bacterial infections, at least in the initial stages. In neonatal maladjustment syndrome (NMS) convulsions it may be up to 40.5°C (105°F)
Subnormal rectal temperature – coma

Total white blood cells (WBC):
    greater than $14 \times 10^9/l$ in septicaemia
    less than $4 \times 10^9/l$ in premature foals
Overwhelming infections
    EHV-1 foals
    combined immunodeficiency disease (CID) foals
Urine from nephritis cases will contain leucocytes, bacteria, protein and
    epithelial cells

Prematurity

Underweight
Soft, pliant ears and lips
Fine, silky coat
Hypoxia – responds to O_2
Increased slope to axis of pastern
Decreased ability to handle renal Na and K
Decreased cortisol
Leucopaenia, neutropaenia
Neutrophil : lymphocyte ratio < 1.0 (instead of > 2.0)

Treatment
Intensive care and supportive therapy:
    nutrition
    prevent sores
    keep dry
    warmth
    oxygen
    monitor vital signs, acid–base electrolyte status, hydration
    broad spectrum antibiotics
    ensure adequate colostrum/plasma

Neonatal conditions

The conditions that affect the neonatal foal are of diverse aetiology and may
be infective or non-infective. The non-infective conditions may present with
gross behavioural disturbances, with developmental abnormality or with
immunological reaction.

It is difficult to diagnose infections in foals because the early clinical signs
are not specific. Infections of the neonatal foal are characterized by common
clinical signs of fever, lethargy, loss of suck reflex, elevated heart and
respiratory rates and a reluctance or inability to stand.

Predisposing factors are chronic endometritis, overcrowded and frequently used foaling boxes, handling of the umbilical cord and premature cutting of the umbilical cord.

Causal organisms of foal infections

Older foals
Bacillus piliformis
Corynebacterium equi
Salmonella
Streptococci

Younger foals
Actinobacillus equuli
β-haemolytic streptococci
Escherichia coli
EHV-1
Klebsiella
Staphylococci

Actinobacillus equuli ('sleepy foal disease', 'shigellosis')

An acute, rapidly fatal infection. The organism is commonly found in the gastrointestinal tract and tissues of adults, with inevitable environmental contamination, and has a predilection for the kidneys, adrenal glands and the brain.

Clinical signs
Initial fever to 39°C (102.5°F)
Depression
Anorexia, ultimately stops sucking
Diarrhoea with mild colic
Convulsions
Uraemia
Coma – 'sleepy foal' which can be aroused but rapidly reverts to a comatose
    state

Diagnosis
From the clinical signs supported by laboratory findings.

Aids to diagnosis
Haematology – total WBC increased
PCV – increased
Blood urea nitrogen – elevated (>20.7 mmol/l)

Urine may contain leucocytes and bacteria, which if present confirm the diagnosis

Treatment
Antibiotics without delay, preferably given in two or three divided doses, parenterally. The therapy should be evaluated against the response obtained. Suggested antibiotics include amoxycillin or trimethoprim and sulphadiazine combination but other penicillins, e.g. ampicillin, cloxacillin or chloramphenicol may be used

Antipyretics

Supportive therapy – dam's plasma given intravenously on two or three occasions at 3-hourly intervals (whole blood if the PCV is < 35%)

Ensure a sufficient intake of milk, best in up to 12 feeds per day at 80 ml/kg bodyweight

Prognosis
Most cases run an acute course and die within 24 hours. Any that survive the first 24 hours may live up to one week and develop septic polyarthritis and renal abscess.

Post-mortem examination
If death occurs within 24 hours there are signs of acute septicaemia with inflammatory foci in the kidneys, liver and lungs, from which the organism can be isolated.

Foals which survive longer than 24 hours have microabscesses in the renal cortex and the joint fluid may be purulent.

Other septicaemias of the young foal

Most commonly seen on the second day, but can appear at any time after birth to the fourth day. The causal organisms tend to have predilection sites in the foal.

S. zooepidemicus	lungs, pleura, peritoneum, joints
E. coli	and umbilicus
Klebsiella	
EHV-1 and cytomegalovirus	lung and liver tissue
Staphylococci	articular and periarticular
Salmonella	tissue, including epiphyses

Clinical signs
Initially:
   dullness

reluctance to feed
normal or slightly raised rectal temperature
Several hours:
elevated temperature to 41°C (106°F) or subnormal
elevated pulse and respiratory rates
pale or injected mucous membranes
rapid dehydration
recumbent
slight jaundiced tinge to sclera
Subsequently:
convulsions
swollen joints
pneumonia

Diagnosis

A septicaemia must always be suspected if any of the clinical signs are seen. It may be possible to differentiate the different stages as the disease progresses. Use the clinical signs supported by laboratory findings.

Aids to diagnosis

Bacteriology: blood culture or isolation of the organism from post-mortem material. Material for a blood culture should be taken before antibiotic therapy is started
Haematology:
reduced RBC and haemoglobin
slow rise in WBC above $10 \times 10^9/l$ with a leucopenia in some cases
PCV falls to 36% then rises to 45% with dehydration

Treatment

Must be started immediately.
The antibiotic must be selected and used before the causal organism has been identified and its sensitivity to antibiotics known. The antibiotic selected must therefore fulfil at least the following criteria:
1 Activity against a broad spectrum of organisms, including both Gram-positive and Gram-negative organisms.
2 A bactericidal agent is preferred which should rapidly achieve high levels in the bloodstream. This inevitably requires the antibiotic to be available in a form suitable for intravenous administration.
3 Good penetration of joints, cartilage, tendon sheaths and into the cerebrospinal fluid (CSF) by the antibiotic, preferably before they are inflamed.
4 If renal function is reduced, sulphonamides and aminoglycosides should be avoided.
Supportive therapy and good nursing.

Prognosis
Poor if a leucopenia is present
The sequel to a septicaemia, if they survive, includes bacteraemic shock, meningitis, pneumonia, growth plate, joint infections and abscessation of internal organs

Post-mortem examination
Mainly non-specific signs typical of a septicaemia – including petechial haemorrhages on serous surfaces, pericarditis, peritonitis and pleurisy. In addition, a suppurative polyarthritis, osteomyelitis and a chondritis of the growth plates may be found.

Septic polyarthritis 'joint ill', 'navel ill'

Many foals have a bacteraemia, due to infection gaining entry through the umbilicus, which does not develop into an acute fatal septicaemia.

In a proportion of foals there is spread to, and localization in, the joints and tendon sheaths. This is from a reservoir of infection, either from an umbilical infection, as a sequel to a septicaemia or from an alimentary tract infection. Infective tenosynovitis can develop from an infection adjacent to the tendon sheath and spread to the joint capsule, or in the reverse direction. A higher incidence of 'joint ill' was found in foals where there was a reduced or delayed intake of colostrum.

Clinical signs
Lameness is a consistent sign
Hot, painful joints, in particular hock, stifle, carpus, in which there is thickening of the joint capsule, synovial distension and oedema of the periarticular tissue
Fever up to 38.5°C (102°F) may be present
A hard/soft swelling, thickening or abscessation of the umbilicus

Diagnosis
From the clinical signs supported by diagnostic aids.

Aids to diagnosis
Arthrocentesis – joint fluid discoloured with leucocytes and fibrin. Elevated total protein, an easy and rapid measurement, and a leucocyte count of $1–50 \times 10^9$/l is diagnostic and invaluable in differentiating an infection from traumatic joint capsule distension. Culture of the synovial fluid is usually negative
Radiography – useful to differentiate infection from traumatic joint capsule distension and to establish the extent of damage to articular or periarticular tissues

Differential diagnosis

Traumatic damage – results in distension of the joint capsule with reduction in the degree of flexion obtained with pain on any movement of the joint. See above

Osteochrondrosis – requires careful radiographic examination to enable a diagnosis where there is a swollen joint with no evidence of inflammation or infection found on examination of the synovial fluid

Treatment

Irreparable damage occurs quickly, probably in less than 24 hours. The treatment must be instituted as rapidly as possible to reduce the severity of damage

Antibiotics – by parenteral injection to control epiphyseal infection and to avoid spread. Intra-articular injection on its own or following joint flushing

Corticosteroids – should be used sparingly on a maximum of one or two occasions

Joint flushing – lavage with 5–10 l of lactated Ringer's or sterile saline previously warmed to body temperature to remove the fibrin and neutrophils. Antibiotics may be infused into the joint following the lavage. (See also Chapter 15)

Prognosis

The prognosis must always be guarded and a worse prognosis given if there is multiple joint involvement, or pronounced lameness which fails to respond to treatment.

Some cases do not respond and euthanasia is indicated for the following cases:

1   Erosion of the cartilage and bone with/without ankylosis.
2   Deformation of the epiphyses.
3   Adhesions between the joint capsule and overlying structures.
4   Humanitarian reasons.

Septicaemic conditions of the older foal

Causal organisms commonly involved:

Bacillus piliformis (Tyzzer's disease)

Rhodococcus equi – see below

Salmonella spp. – see below

Septic polyarthritis is also seen in foals up to four months of age and is caused by a number of organisms including

S. typhimurium and *R. equi,* the latter having been isolated from epiphyseal abscesses

Tyzzer's disease

An acute hepatitis affecting foals of 2–6 weeks of age caused by a spore-bearing bacillus (*B. piliformis*). The disease has a sporadic incidence with infection thought to be by ingestion of spores present in the bedding or faeces of horses.

Clinical signs

Peracute form
Foal can be found dead

Acute form
Extreme depression
Collapse
Fever may be present
Jaundice may be present
Convulsions later
Coma and death

Diagnosis

Most frequently made on post-mortem examination as the foal appears normal before a short, terminal illness.

Differential diagnosis

Severe anaemia – foal is unwell the day before death
Congenital EHV-1 – foal dies before two weeks of age
Acute liver necrosis from poisoning – very rare

Post-mortem examination

Grossly enlarged liver with pale foci which on histopathological examination show as multiple areas of focal necrosis surrounded by acute inflammatory cell infiltration. Liver cells at the edge of the lesion show the characteristic intracytoplasmic bacilli or spores if special stains, e.g. Giemsa and Levaditti, are used.

Respiratory tract infections

Foals (and yearlings) are particularly prone to respiratory tract infections, especially in studs and yards which have a high turnover of mares and foals. Any horse that arrives with an infection or suspected infection must be isolated immediately. The commonest presenting sign is a rhinitis, frequently of multiple aetiology.

Viruses involved
Influenza virus
EHV
Adenovirus (CID in Arabian foals)
Rhinovirus

Bacteria involved
As a primary infection – *C. equi*
Commonly as secondary infections – Streptococci
Staphylococci
E.coli

Endoparasites involved
Parascaris equorum
Migrating strongyle larvae

Upper respiratory tract disease of foals

The clinical signs with viral infection are as described in Chapter 1. In addition, influenza and adenovirus infection in foals may cause a proliferating pneumonia with an increased possibility of acute or chronic bronchopneumonia.

Clinical signs
Nasal discharge: initially serous, rapidly becomes profuse, mucopurulent
    and may persist
Pneumonia:
    increased temperature
    dyspnoea
    acute or chronic bronchopneumonia

Diagnosis
From the clinical signs.

Diagnostic aids
Bacteriological examination of nasal swabs
Virus isolation from nasopharyngeal swabs
Serology – may assist retrospectively

Treatment
In all cases of pneumonia and when there is a persistent nasal discharge,
    antibiotic therapy, e.g. penicillins or sulphonamide-potentiated tri-
    methoprim products, is indicated and should be continued until after the
    clinical signs abate

Clean blocked nostrils
Apply petroleum jelly at the first signs of 'scalding' of the nares and muzzle
Mucolytics, e.g. Sputolosin (Boehringer Ingelheim), may be helpful

Prognosis
Good in the majority of cases
Chronic pulmonary damage, with possible abscess formation

Prevention
It is not possible in a stud or yard to prevent upper respiratory tract (URT) infections. Contact with stud mares provides a 'natural' vaccine by the repeated challenge of EHV-1 infection.

Yearlings are best exposed to yard infections to allow the infections to run their course prior to them being put into training.

Foals should be vaccinated against equine influenza from three months of age.

Lower respiratory tract disease of foals

Bacterial pneumonia
Frequently there is a history of intercurrent disease, in particular URT tract infections, stress or debility associated with the onset.

Clinical signs
Depression, lethargy, cessation of sucking
Elevated temperature
Increased pulse rate
Increased respiratory rate and effort, even laboured in severe cases
Moist, harsh cough
Abnormal lung sounds possibly with fluid line
Cyanosis may be present

Diagnosis
Initially from the clinical signs.

Aids to diagnosis
Haematology – useful in monitoring progression of the disease and response to treatment
Tracheal wash – identify the causal organism, initially by direct smear with bacterial culture and antibiotic sensitivity tests following
Radiography – assessment of consolidation or abscessation
Thoracocentesis – if there is a detectable fluid line, with laboratory examination of any fluid withdrawn

Differential diagnosis

S. zooepidemicus is most commonly found

C. equi is less commonly found

Pasteurella/Actinobacillus are found but the exact significance of their presence is unknown

Staphylococci, *Klebsiella, Salmonella, E. coli* and *Pseudomonas* are usually associated with a bacteraemia such as 'navel ill' or 'joint ill'

Treatment

Penicillin is the drug of first choice as the commonest respiratory pathogen is β-haemolytic streptococcus which is sensitive to penicillin

(N.B. If ampicillin is to be used it must be in the form of the sodium salt)

The choice of antibiotic may change following antibiotic sensitivity tests or if there is no response to the antibiotic currently used

In severe cases oxygen may be beneficial

Mucolytics, e.g. Sputolosin (Boehringer Ingelheim)

Bronchodilators

A single dose of corticosteroid, with/without diuretics, is indicated if the oedema appears to be killing the foal faster than the bacteria

Prognosis

Always give a guarded prognosis. An early diagnosis with prompt, vigorous treatment, for a sufficiently long period of time, will improve the prognosis

The resting respiratory rate is a good guide to the eventual outcome – if it stays high the prognosis is poor

A continued high total white cell count with a degenerative shift to the left and a foal that continues with depression and anorexia indicates an unfavourable outcome. Such foals fail to thrive and become 'poor doers'

Rhodococcus equi infection – respiratory form

This infectious disease of foals 2–3 months old, and sometimes older, is insidious in onset with pulmonary changes well advanced before clinical signs appear. The condition is sporadic and may be restricted to particular farms. Mode of entry of the organism is thought to be by inhalation or ingestion as the organism is thought to survive in the soil. It has been suggested that migrating parasitic larvae may carry the infection through the body.

The respiratory form is thought to be a sequel to the alimentary form, if present.

History

One of failure to thrive, with a persistent cough.

Clinical signs
Increased respiratory rate with dyspnoea
Fever of 39–41°C (102.5–106°F)
Cough
Mucopurulent nasal discharge
Lung sounds – moist rales with areas of dullness
Abdominal pain – if concurrent alimentary involvement
Joint ill cases – *R. equi* can be found in the epiphyseal abscesses

Diagnosis
Very difficult to confirm a diagnosis of *R. equi* in the living foal. A provisional diagnosis may be made on a persistent high temperature, signs of pneumonia and failure to respond to antibiotic therapy.

Aids to diagnosis
Tracheal wash – the positive identification of the *R. equi* organisms should be attempted despite the difficulty in isolation of this organism. May be false negatives as the organism is intracellular
Nasal swabs – culture of the organism from nasal swabs is less successful than from a tracheal wash material
Radiography – can be carried out in an attempt to identify thick-walled abscesses. Interpretation can be difficult and equipment of sufficient power must be available
Haematology – will indicate a chronic infective process. Plasma fibrinogen concentration increased

Treatment
Penicillin and gentamicin have been suggested at high doses every 8 or 12 hours. Once the organism is in the abscess, the antibiotics do not seem to penetrate the thick wall of the abscess. Other antibiotics, erythromycin, neomycin and rifampicin, are effective against *R. equi* organisms *in vitro*. Erythromycin and rifampicin, both highly lipid-soluble, are able to enter and become concentrated in macrophages and neutrophils and kill intracellular bacteria. Although very expensive, erythromycin 25 mg/kg t.i.d. and rifampicin 5 mg/kg b.i.d. per os, until the chest radiographs and plasma fibrinogen return to normal, have been successful in some cases.

Treatment is unrewarding and has little effect on the course of the condition.

Prognosis
The respiratory form can develop rapidly with the foal dying within ten days. Other cases continue for weeks with a mortality rate of 80%, either dying naturally or having to be euthanased. (See also alimentary form, p. 80.)

Pneumocystis carinii

Pneumocystis carinii has recently been confirmed as a fungus although its life cycle is uncertain. Reports are rare in horses, most having been in Arab foals suffering from CID. (It is currently the most common opportunistic infection in human patients with acquired immunodeficiency syndrome.)

Clinical signs

Sudden onset pyrexia and dyspnoea which is unresponsive to therapy. Death is within five days. Diagnosis is based on presence of interstitial pneumonia supported by histopathology

Alimentary tract disease of foals

Meconium impaction and retention

Normally the dark green/black meconium is passed in the first 4–96 hours of life. There then follows the normal yellow faeces which result from the ingestion and digestion of colostrum and milk. The consistency of meconium varies. Hard faecal pellets cause the impaction of the colon or rectum.

Clinical signs

Straining or squatting

Abdominal pain – foal repeatedly looks at its flanks. An apparent discomfort increases to abdominal pain when the foal sucks. The foal may roll on to its back with its legs in the air

Increased pulse and respiratory rate

May also stop sucking

Impacted mass found in the pelvis on rectal examination

Diagnosis

From the clinical signs supported by the history of the foal passing very little, if any, meconium.

Differential diagnosis

Bladder rupture – urine only passed in small quantities with abdominal distension from fluid (which can be confirmed by percussion and abdominal paracentesis)

Other causes of intestinal obstruction – usually found if the foal continues to deteriorate, despite treatment, and an exploratory laparotomy is carried out

Tetanus – the first sign of tetanus in a foal is often constipation

Treatment
300–500 ml liquid paraffin by stomach tube

Enema – if a soapy water enema is used it must be by gravity, not administered under pressure

Analgesia – 5–10 ml pethidine 5% solution intramuscularly

Restrain the foal to avoid injury

Gentle digital manipulation, although possible, should be avoided as it may exacerbate the condition and may even perforate the rectal wall

Surgical removal may be necessary if very dry impacted meconium is present in the colon

Prognosis
Meconium impaction seldom causes death but intestinal rupture (and rectal rupture) with peritonitis can occur.

Diarrhoea

Diarrhoea is a common clinical problem in foals, with a high incidence in foals up to five months of age. Most have a mild diarrhoea at least once before weaning and recover spontaneously. It is probable that several factors combine in many cases to produce the clinical signs of diarrhoea.

The aetiology includes nutritional, bacterial, viral and parasitic causes.

Nutritional diarrhoeas
Various dietary causes may exist and include:
1   Changes in milk composition.
2   Excessive milk intake.
3   Ingestion of foreign materials.

Changes in milk composition
Diarrhoea occurs at 7–10 days of age when the mare is in oestrus and is well recognized as the 'foal heat scour'. Although regarded by many veterinarians as being physiological, there is no evidence of a correlation between the milk composition and the onset of diarrhoea.

Clinical signs
A mild, usually transient, diarrhoea is the common clinical sign.

Diagnosis
A definite diagnosis is seldom made, nor is it required in the majority of cases.

Treatment
Antibiotic therapy should be avoided
Reduce milk intake using a muzzle
Provide oral electrolyte/glucose solutions in the drinking water
Oral administration of intestinal absorbants, e.g. kaolin – of questionable
　　value

Prognosis
The above treatment(s) will assist what is probably a spontaneous recovery.
The foal must be monitored carefully for evidence of a more serious attack of
diarrhoea developing, caused by a virulent pathogen.

Excessive milk intake
Foals with persistent or recurring diarrhoea may respond to reduction of
milk intake or early weaning. This continual diarrhoea may be due to a
lactose intolerance following an acute or chronic enteritis, possibly of viral
origin, resulting in a malabsorption of sugars.

Diagnosis
A provisional diagnosis can be made from the failure of the foal to recover
spontaneously from an episode of mild diarrhoea or from repeated episodes
of diarrhoea. The use of the oral lactose test may assist in confirming the
diagnosis.

Treatment
Change the foal to a non-lactose diet with supportive therapy
Response to this treatment will assist in confirming the diagnosis

Prognosis
Good for a marked clinical improvement in the majority of cases.

Ingestion of foreign materials
Coprophagia – is common in foals of 2–5 weeks of age. It is thought to 'seed'
the gut with bacteria, only causing diarrhoea if the faeces contain enter-
opathogenic bacteria.
　　Fibre is necessary for the development of the foal's large intestine. The
alimentary tract is, however, very sensitive to changes in dietary composition
and increasing quantities of roughage ingested may precipitate a digestive
disorder, in particular if the material is indigestible.
　　Ingestion of bedding or irritant materials, such as disinfectants, may lead
to diarrhoea. The availability should be avoided with an improvement in
husbandry if necessary. Removal of the cause is sufficient, and the foal will
recover spontaneously.

Bacterial diarrhoeas

A significant number of diarrhoeas in other species are associated with a mixed infection. In foals a mixed infection with rotavirus and *S. typhimurium* has been described and it is likely that others will be identified.

Organisms involved:

1 *E. coli.*
2 *Salmonella* spp.
3 *R. equi*
4 *Campylobacter* spp.
5 *Clostridium perfringens.*

Enteric colibacillosis

It is possible that many cases of diarrhoea in foals are due to this organism. The challenge presented to foals from *E.coli* organisms is less than in other species due to the lower stocking rates, cleaning of foaling boxes between foalings and the greater individual care to ensure adequate colostral intake by the foal.

Clinical signs

Generally a mild diarrhoea
May progress to a more severe diarrhoea with dehydration, lethargy and
    reluctance to suck

Diagnosis

Will probably not be diagnosed as an *E. coli* diarrhoea. Specific *E. coli* serotypes have not been recognized in foals.

Treatment

Symptomatic treatment with the use of antibiotics if necessary.

Prognosis

Good with a low mortality rate.

Salmonella spp.

In diarrhoea caused by *Salmonella* infection in foals, *S. typhimurium* is the causal organism in 75% of the cases. Clinical signs are due to the activation of a latent infection by stress or by the ingestion of massive numbers of the bacteria.

Clinical signs

Depressed foal
Injected mucous membranes

Fever to 42°C (108°F)
Elevated pulse and respiratory rates
Abdominal pain
Profuse watery faeces with a fetid odour which may contain blood and
    mucus
Rapid dehydration
Significant neutropenia develops rapidly

Diagnosis
From the clinical signs, in particular the type of diarrhoea in a depressed,
very ill foal and the rapid development of a significant neutropenia.

Treatment
Sulphonamide/trimethoprim combinations intravenously
Chloramphenicol intravenously
Fluids, electrolytes or plasma intravenously

Prognosis
Very poor as there is a sudden onset and rapid development of clinical signs
followed by circulatory collapse and death.

N.B. This a zoonotic disease and staff must take every care to avoid
infection. Precautions must be taken to avoid spread to other parts of the
yard and subsequently the box must be cleaned and disinfected thoroughly.

Rhodococcus equi – alimentary form
In the alimentary form the organism tends to localize in the intestinal wall
and the mesenteric lymph nodes. *R. equi* organisms have been isolated in
mesenteric lymph nodes of apparently normal foals.

Clinical signs
Insidious onset with weight loss
Abdominal pain
Diarrhoea (may not be present in all cases) can be acute, chronic or inter-
    mittent
Respiratory form may be present concurrently – see Respiratory tract
    infections, p. 75

Diagnosis
Difficult to diagnose except by exploratory laparotomy. The presence of *R.
equi* organisms in a foal's liquid faeces is highly suggestive and in Britain can
be considered to confirm the diagnosis. In Australia the organism appears to
be a normal member of the equine faecal flora.

Treatment

Considerable variation in antibiotic sensitivity is found but the organism is usually sensitive to neomycin, erythromycin, rifampicin and gentamicin. High doses are recommended every 8–12 hours over a prolonged period.

Prognosis

Poor if not hopeless. The response to treatment is disappointing as the lesions are well advanced before treatment is instituted (see also *R. equi* respiratory form, p. 78).

Post-mortem examination

Gross thickening of the intestinal wall and enlargement of abdominal lymph nodes. In chronic cases there is mucosal necrosis and ulceration with villous atrophy. The lymph nodes are oedematous and contain bacteria-laden macrophages.

Campylobacter spp.

Campylobacter jejuni subspecies *coli* has been found in the faeces of foals with diarrhoea. As cultural techniques improve, the incidence diagnosed will probably increase. Although its significance is unknown, the importance of *Campylobacter* species infection must not be underestimated.

Clinical signs

Diarrhoea – probably a mild form in most cases
Colic (present in all reported cases)

Diagnosis

The presence of diarrhoea with the isolation of *Campylobacter* spp. from the faeces.

Treatment

The use of erythromycin and tylosin appears to eliminate the organism from the faeces, and they should be considered as suitable antibiotics in the treatment of foals with diarrhoea from which the organism has been isolated.

Prognosis

Presumed to be good in most cases. *Campylobacter* has been isolated from gastric and duodenal ulcers at post-mortem examination, which, with a report that up to 30% of foal deaths are associated with gastric and duodenal ulceration and a similar percentage with diarrhoea, suggests that the true role of the organism is at present underestimated.

N.B. The danger to handlers of affected foals requires appropriate hygienic practices to be instituted.

Clostridium perfringens types **B** and **C**

Can cause sporadic cases of enterotoxaemia in 1–2-day-old foals with a stud outbreak possible.

Clinical signs

Peracute form
    Foal may be found dead
Acute form
    Severe systemic illness
    Acute onset depression
    Fever of 39–40°C (102.5–104°F)
    Tachycardia
    Blood-stained faeces

Diagnosis

The clinical signs with abnormally high levels of *C. perfringens* organisms in the faeces are considered diagnostic. More commonly the diagnosis is made by the presence of enterotoxins in the gut at post-mortem examination.

Treatment

Prompt administration of antibiotics with intravenous fluids may save the foal
Lamb dysentery antiserum should be given prophylactically, at birth preferably, to prevent further cases in the stud

Prognosis

Very poor.

Viral diarrhoeas

The incidence of viral diarrhoea in foals is unknown but an increasing number of reports suggest that they are a major enteric pathogen of foals.

Rotavirus infection

Clinically the infection may range from mild to severe.

Clinical signs

Pyrexia
Depression
Anorexia
Teeth grinding
Abdominal pain
Watery diarrhoea within 24 hours of onset of illness

Diagnosis

On clinical signs, with confirmation from virus isolation
Gastrointestinal tract ulceration may be present

Treatment

Spontaneous recovery is possible or symptomatic treatment may be necessary
Antibiotic therapy should be considered if there is a secondary bacterial infection
Sucralfate/ranitidine if gastroduodenal ulcer suspected

Prognosis

Most cases recover within 48–72 hours.

Coronavirus and adenovirus infection

Both groups of viruses have been detected in foals with diarrhoea, but the significance of these agents in foal enteric disease has yet to be determined.

In other species, coronavirus is probably the second most common viral agent, but there are few reports at present of enteric infection of foals with coronavirus.

Adenoviruses are common respiratory pathogens but up to 50% of foals affected with adenovirus type 1 have diarrhoea.

Parasitic diarrhoeas

Strongyloides westeri: foals are often infected in the first few days of life due to the ingestion of infective larvae in the mare's milk which become patent by two weeks of age

Strongyle spp: mixed infections may cause diarrhoea once the foal starts to ingest significant amounts of grass. This would probably produce cases late in the grazing season
See Chapter 6 for more detail

Eimeria leuckarti oöcysts have been found in faeces of foals as young as 15 days of age. Oöcysts have been shed intermittently for about four months

Control of infectious diarrhoea in foals

The role of individual pathogens in foal diarrhoea is of limited importance when considering prevention/control, as most of the diarrhoeas are of multiple aetiology. The role of stress in clinical diarrhoea is uncertain.

Colostral antibodies have an important role in the prevention of diarrhoea and high antibody levels can be obtained by ensuring that foals ingest and absorb adequate colostrum in the first 24 hours of life.

General cleanliness in the yard and in particular of the foaling accommodation is most important in the prevention of foal diarrhoeas.

In all mild cases of foal diarrhoea the owner should take the rectal temperature three times daily and notify any change in severity of the diarrhoea or the foal's demeanour.

Gastroduodenal ulceration

The cause of gastroduodenal ulceration has not been established but is associated with stress and the use of non-steroidal anti-inflammatory drugs. It has been suggested that ulceration may be related to, or follow, disease, e.g. rotavirus infection. May be associated with strictures in the duodenum.

Clinical signs
Range from those associated with perforation giving peritonitis; colic following suckle; anorexia; depression; to a lack of apparent clinical signs.
Seen from one day to four months.

Diagnosis
From clinical signs, supported by endoscopy and radiography with contrast media
Paracentesis will be normal unless ulcer perforated

Differential diagnosis
Pharyngeal/oesophageal dysfunctions
Cleft palate
Other causes of abdominal pain

Treatment
Oral protectives: bismuth subsalicylate or sucralfate
Antacids:

ranitidine	2.2 mg/kg per os b. to t.i.d.
	0.5 mg/kg i.v. q.i.d.
cimetidine	6.6 mg/kg per os t.i.d.
	2.0 mg/kg i.v. q.i.d.

Treat as above for at least four weeks to allow healing
Supportive:
 nursing
 fluids
 gastric decompression if necessary
 surgical for strictures

Neonatal maladjustment syndrome (NMS)

Also known as 'Wanderers', 'Barkers', 'Dummies' or 'convulsive foals'. It is mainly seen in thoroughbreds and the signs develop within the first 24 hours of life and commonly in the first hour after birth.

Clinical signs
Variable and may consist of some or all of the following:
1   Convulsions – clonic or generalized following or alternating with periods of coma.
2   Foal may appear blind.
    Asymmetrical pupillary apertures common.
    Scleral and retinal haemorrhages.
3   Loss of suck reflex.
4   Exaggerated response to handling.
    Violent movements when recumbent.
    Inability to stand.
    Aimless wandering around box.
    Opisthotonus.
    Tail held upright.
5   Sneezing.
    Vocalization.
    Clinical signs may last 30 days. During the recovery phase there is a definite sequence – coma, ability to get up and stand, then return of auditory and visual awareness before the ability to suck.

Diagnosis
The presence of the most consistent signs (convulsions, inability to suck and ocular changes) and the age of the foal.

Treatment
Supportive and symptomatic:
• Prevent exhaustion and trauma to the foal
• Feed by stomach tube (80 ml/kg/day), including colostrum, and ensure dehydration does not develop
• Keep warm
• Counteract acidosis – 5–10 ml of 5% sodium bicarbonate i.v.
• Counteract hypoxia – oxygen
• Control convulsions – no noise in and around the stable
• anticonvulsant – phenytoin i.v., i.m., orally: loading dose 5–10 mg/kg then 1–5 mg/kg every 2–4 hours, reducing to every 6–12 hours – after 12 hours depending on the severity of the convulsions
• Broad spectrum antibiotic therapy during the course of the condition

- Cardiac failure – digoxin 0.06 mg/kg divided into six doses over two days (t.i.d.), then 0.01 mg/kg divided b.i.d.

Prognosis

A poor or guarded prognosis is given initially which is modified on appearance of the recovery sequence.

Combined immunodeficiency disease (CID)

Disease of Arabian/part-Arabian foals, inherited as an autosomal recessive trait, which are unable to be immunocompetent.

Affected foals appear normal at first. When passive maternal antibody levels decline the foals are immunodeficient. They are then highly susceptible to a variety of infectious diseases, in particular respiratory disease (a true viral pneumonia with adenovirus infection). No effective treatment.

Male and female offspring are equally affected and do not live to breeding age. Do not breed from known carriers.

Neonatal isoerythrolysis

Intravascular and extravascular haemolysis occurs in the foal due to post-partum absorption of alloantigens concentrated in colostrum. While it is more common in mares that have had previous foals, the primary sensitization could be from prior blood transfusion.

Clinical signs

Normal at birth with clinical signs eight hours to five days *post-partum*
Lethargy
Weakness
Loss of suck reflex
Yawning
Pale to icteric with tachycardia possible, haemoglobinaemia after 24–36 hours

Diagnosis

A total red blood cell count of < 4 000 000/ml and haemoglobin < 7 g/dl is very suggestive. Confirmed by agglutination and direct Coombs' test.

Treatment

Do not stress foal
If foal is less than 36 hours old, withhold dam's colostrum and give supplement
If PCV less than 10%, or less than 15% and falling rapidly, transfuse:
- Donor Aa and Oa negative

- RBCs from dam washed three times with saline, giving 1–2 litres
- Can do exchange transfusion giving 5 litres and bleeding 5 litres
- Supportive therapy

Prevention
Test mare's serum in last two weeks of pregnancy against known erythrocyte alloantigens. If positive, withhold colostrum and supplement from elsewhere or prevent nursing until known if foal erythrocytes will be affected.

Recommended further reading

Rossdale P.D. & Ricketts S.W. (1980) *Equine Stud Farm Medicine* (2nd edn). Baillière, Tindall, London.

6 / Internal parasites

Internal parasites of the horse in Britain include:
Large strongyles
    Strongylus vulgaris
    Strongylus edentatus
Small strongyles
    Trichonema species (*Cythanostomum* species)
Threadworms
    Strongyloides westeri
Lungworms
    Dictyocaulus arnfieldi
Tapeworms
    Anoplocephela species
    Echinococcus granulosus
Flukes
    Fasciola hepatica
Bot larvae
    Gastrophilus intestinalis
Pin worm
    Oxyuris equi

The most important group of parasites in the horse is the strongyles. *Parascaris equorum* is of special importance in the foal. All horses are parasitized to a certain degree; the development of clinical disease will depend on the age of the horse, nature of the worm burden, exposure to infection and the type of control programme.

Strongyles

Naturally acquired infections are always by ingestion of third stage larvae (L3) during grazing.

The larvae will have developed from eggs passed in the faeces of grazing horses. The numbers of pasture larvae increase from the spring through the summer and autumn, in particular when the conditions are warm and moist.

Strongylus vulgaris

Life cycle
The third stage (infective) larvae penetrate the mucosa of the small and large

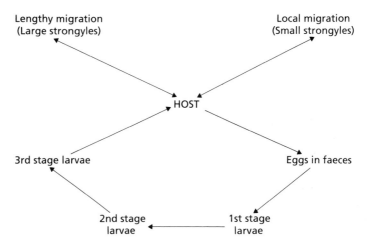

Fig. 6.1 Life cycle of strongyles.

intestines, moult to fourth stage larvae and penetrate the arterioles by seven days post-infection. There is a migration to reach the mesenteric root by 21 days post-infection, development of the larvae to fifth stage larvae and return to the intestine through the lumen of the blood vessels. At the serosal surface of the intestine the larvae are surrounded by nodules, with subsequent rupture of these nodules releasing the young adults into the gut lumen where they become sexually mature. The full life cycle takes at least five and up to seven months. See Fig. 6.1.

Clinical signs

Foals
Massive larval invasion:
- Severe depression, sudden in onset
- Colic
- Death

Small numbers of larvae ingested:
- Dullness
- Anorexia
- Pyrexia
- Abdominal pain

Yearlings and older horses
Weight loss or failure to thrive
Chronic wasting with anaemia, hypoproteinaemia, intermittent colic and periodic soft faeces
Protein-losing gastroenteropathy with malabsorption and low serum albumin and high β-globulin levels

Recurrent colic and vascular damage which could lead to a 'surgical colic'
Cerebrospinal nematodiasis from the aberrant migration of larvae through
    the CNS which gives variable neurological signs

Strongylus edentatus

Life cycle
The infective third stage larvae following ingestion penetrate the caecum and
right ventral colon and reach the liver via the portal bloodstream within two
days. Migration in the liver is over about 7–9 weeks, producing white foci
consisting of necrotic eosinophils. They leave the liver at the hepatic liga-
ments and pass to the subperitoneal tissue where they cause the formation of
haemorrhagic nodules. After about three months and a moult to fifth stage
larvae, migration to the intestinal wall takes place where large haemorrhagic
nodules are formed which will rupture, releasing the immature adults into the
lumen of the bowel. The prepatent period is about 11 months.

Clinical signs

Foals
Poor growth, anaemia and debility with possible diarrhoea

Older horses
Weight loss or failure to thrive
Peritonitis – from the fibrinous adhesions within the abdomen

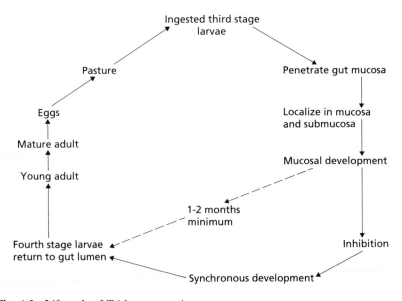

Fig. 6.2 Life cycle of *Trichonema* species.

Liver dysfunction – from the migratory phase or from the granulomas in the
    liver and pancreas occasionally produced by the parasites which occlude
    the bile duct
This parasite may be implicated in horses presented with, in addition, a
    hypoalbuminaemia and elevated γ GT levels

Trichonema species

Life cycle
Migration of the larval stages is limited to the wall of the caecum and colon
although some larvae may penetrate the small intestine (see Fig. 6.2). The
prepatent period is probably from 42 days with significant numbers of eggs
not being found until 56–70 days post-infection. Foals may have patent
infections from 6–9 weeks of age.

Clinical signs
Clinical cases are usually seen between December and May
Poor performance
Weight loss with appetite maintained
Diarrhoea – sudden onset with a chronic course
Oedema of the limbs – hypoalbuminaemia
Colic and pyrexia may or may not be present
Numerous red fourth stage larvae in the faeces or on the surface of the
    disposable sleeve following rectal examination

Aids to diagnosis
Haematology – neutrophilia common, the degree of increase is related to the
    severity of the problem
Eosinophilia in some cases, frequently counts are low or negative
Blood chemistry:
    hypoalbuminaemia
    elevated β (+α) globulins common
Faeces – egg counts usually low (0–200 e.p.g.)

Diagnosis of mixed strongyles infections
1 History:
    pasture size and the number of horses
    length of time grazed
    standard of pasture management
    worming history and anthelmintic used.
2 Clinical examination – reveals few significant diagnostic abnormalities,
other than *Trichonema* fourth stage larvae in the faeces or an enlarged
anterior mesenteric artery. It has been suggested that colic is the single most
common clinical manifestation of strongyle infections.

3 Faecal examination – only an accurate test of the presence of mature adult infestation. A heavy infestation of inhibited larvae or migratory larvae may be present despite a negative faecal egg count.

4 Blood examination:

Anaemia – normocytic, normochromic

Eosinophilia – useful if present but there may be a normal eosinophil count despite a heavy infestation

Leucocytosis due to a neutrophilia

Hypoalbuminaemia

Elevated (alpha and beta) globulins

Treatment

Anthelmintic therapy using a broad spectrum anthelmintic – see list in Chapter 14. Not all anthelmintic preparations are larvicidal and some have different dose rates and routines for the elimination of different species and stages of worms.

Control

Anthelmintics

With drugs which, at normal dose rates, are not effective against migrating larvae or developing *Trichonema* larvae, the minimum interval will be four weeks. With drugs which have larvicidal activity, the interval may be up to eight weeks.

Spring/summer treatments are particularly important for the control of strongyle parasites in the adult horse.

Avoid anthelmintic resistance (at least eight species of cyathostome worms have developed benzimidazole resistance). Anthelmintic treatment for all new arrivals, or returning mares, followed by isolation for two days before joining the herd with a non-benzimidazole anthelmintic to reduce pasture contamination with benzimidazole-resistant worms. Ivermectin, oxibendazole and pyrantel have consistently given good results against benzimidazole resistant small strongyles.

Stable and pasture management

Worm all foals from six weeks of age

Worm mares before they go into the foaling boxes

Keep the boxes clean with frequent removal of faeces

Alternate grazing with cattle and sheep

Remove dung from fields or break up the dung to allow desiccation

Parascaris equorum

An important nematode of foals. Up to 60% of foals are infected compared with 10% of mature horses. Female worms produce thousands of eggs daily which may lead to rapid and persistent contamination of the environment. The eggs have a three-layered shell which can remain viable for many years if the environmental temperature is less than 10°C. Marked resistance commonly develops by 6–12 months of age, with a concurrent decrease in the number of eggs excreted.

Life cycle
The thick-shelled egg, with a sticky outer layer, is passed in the faeces and develops into the infective second stage within the egg in 10–14 days. On ingestion, the egg hatches and the larvae penetrate the intestinal wall, reaching the liver within 48 hours, where they remain for several days. The larvae reach the lungs 7–14 days later, and after reaching the major airways are coughed up and swallowed, with the return to the intestine where growth is completed. The prepatent period is 12–15 weeks. (See Fig. 6.3.)

Clinical signs
Weight loss or lack of liveweight gain despite a good appetite; this becomes
     more marked as the infection develops
Poor coat
Colic

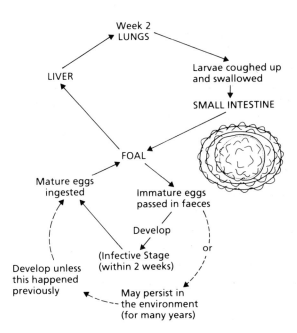

Fig. 6.3 Life cycle of *Parascaris equorum*.

Nervous disturbances
Death due to intestinal rupture or intestinal impaction has been reported

Respiratory form
Coincides with the migration phase and occurs during the third and fourth
  weeks post-infection
Frequent coughing
Grey-white nasal discharge
Copious mucus in the major airways
Fever may be present
Other pathogens may exacerbate the clinical signs

Diagnosis
From the clinical signs supported by the presence of ascarid worm eggs in
the faeces. The history of the premises, in particular parasite control measures, is of assistance in reaching an early diagnosis.

Aids to diagnosis
Faecal examination – eggs first appear in the faeces at about 11–12 weeks
  and have been found in foals of 80 days of age. Negative results only
  eliminate the possibility of a patent infection and the number of eggs in
  the faeces does not accurately reflect the degree of parasitism
Haematology – an eosinophilia may be present between ten and 40 days
  post-infection but is not specific for parascariasis

Treatment
Piperazine citrate at 200 mg/kg bodyweight
Modern broad spectrum anthelmintics

Control

Anthelmintic treatment
All mares should be wormed two days before entering the foaling box
Foals should be dosed at six weeks of age and every four weeks thereafter
  until at least 12 months of age and preferably longer

Management
Pasture management – as described earlier for strongyles. It is important
  that foals are allowed to graze the least contaminated pastures and certainly avoid pastures contaminated by foals of the previous year if at all
  possible
Stable management – foaling boxes should be cleaned and disinfected
  between mares

Mare – wash the udder following the pre-foaling worming to remove any
ascarid eggs which could be ingested by the foal when sucking

Foals – weigh foals regularly and suspect *Parascaris* infection if the foal shows
reduced weight gain or weight loss

Strongyloides westeri

The infective larvae enter the foal either in the mare's milk (from four days
after parturition) or by penetration of the skin: the former route is probably of greater importance. Patent infections of foals develop in two weeks.

Peak egg production is at 8–9 weeks post-infection, which then falls away
with the foal free of infection by six months of age

Clinical signs

Yellowish persistent diarrhoea in foals of 2–4 weeks of age

Lesions may occur (rarely) following percutaneous infection with irritation,
roughening and thickening of the skin

Diagnosis

Diarrhoea with large numbers of thin shelled, larvulated *Strongyloides* eggs in
the faeces

The diarrhoea should be differentiated from bacterial and nutritional scours

Treatment

Thiabendazole and ivermectin at normal dose rates

Oxibendazole at twice the normal dose rate

Fenbendazole at six times the normal dose rate

Oxyuris equi

A white to grey thick-bodied worm. The females migrate to the rectum and
lay their eggs on the perineum. Infection occurs when eggs that have been
rubbed off fall on to feed or water.

Clinical signs

Intense irritation causing restlessness and rubbing against any projection

Hair loss at base of the tail and possible thickening of the skin or even
rupture with secondary bacterial infection

Diagnosis

A clinical pruritus with eggs found in samples taken from the perianal region,
either with sticky acetate tape or scrapings from the perianal region

The eggs are not passed in the faeces

Treatment

Piperazine at 200 mg/kg bodyweight is effective against adults

Modern broad spectrum anthelmintics are highly effective against adult and immature infections

Wash the perianal region and apply antiseptic cream or if necessary an ointment containing local anaesthetic

Dictyocaulus arnfieldi

See Chapter 1.

Anoplocephela perfoliota

The only common tapeworm found in British horses. Infection occurs when horses ingest forage mites, the intermediate hosts. Their pathogenicity is not understood although colic, unthriftiness and diarrhoea have been attributed to severe infestations.

Treatment

Prophylactic treatment is not considered necessary

Niclosamide at 200–300 mg/kg bodyweight and pyrantel at 38 mg/kg, twice the dose rate for routine worming, are the most useful drugs at present

Globidium leuckarti

See 'Parasitic diarrhoea', p. 38.

Echinococcus granulosus

An incidence of up to 60% has been reported from surveys of horses in the UK, with dogs the most likely definitive host of the disease. The horse does not appear to be involved in the hydatidosis cycle affecting humans.

   Clinical manifestations of the disease are rare, with massive infections found in apparently healthy horses at slaughter.

Control

Break the horse-hound cycle by not feeding affected lungs and liver to dogs and routinely treat all at-risk dogs for *Echinococcus* infection.

Fasciola hepatica

Experimental infection of horses indicates a pronounced resistance to infection.

Clinical signs
Clinical disease is unusual, but the following signs have been reported:
- Weight loss
- Increased appetite
- Lethargy
- Poor performance

Diagnosis
Demonstration of ova in the faeces confirms the diagnosis

Treatment
Oxyclonazide at 15 ml/50 kg bodyweight up to a maximum of 100 ml, or
10% w/v triclabendazole at 12 mg/kg.

Gastrophilus intestinalis

Life cycle
The adult flies are active in July to September. They deposit the yellow/
orange eggs typically on the legs but also the lower abdomen and shoulders
of the horse. The eggs hatch after about one week in response to licking and
biting by the horse and the larvae enter the mouth and migrate to the stomach. After about ten months the larvae pass out with the faeces and pupate
on the soil before hatching as adult flies in 3–5 weeks.

Bots are thought to be of little clinical significance but the adult flies
annoy the horse.

Control
Grooming – frequent removal of the eggs with special 'bot combs'–insec-
    ticidal solutions sponged on the body areas where bot flies lay their eggs
Anthelmintic treatment – should be administered after the first frosts have
    killed all the adult flies
Normal anthelmintics are not effective and ivermectin or an organophos-
    phate agent must be used. The latter should not be given to horses which
    are ill for other reasons or have liver damage

7 / Skin diseases

The loss of hair may be the first sign to the owner that a problem exists. This loss of hair may be associated with a pruritus and abnormal behaviour. Skin problems must be regarded seriously, in particular with a show horse.

Alopecia

Alopecia occurs when there is a complete or partial loss of hair and is classified as:

Cicatrical alopecia – this is permanent as there is a complete lack of hair follicles with replacement fibrosis. It occurs as a sequel to third degree burns, deep-seated pyodermas, exposure of the skin to caustic chemicals or as the sequel to severe cutaneous injury.

Non-cicatrical alopecia – occurs more frequently, the most common cause being self-inflicted trauma. In a pruritic dermatosis the alopecia is secondary to the cause of the pruritus, which must be established

Vitiligo

This is characterized by the appearance of depigmentation spots or areas on the skin of the horse. The aetiology is either unknown (idiopathic vitiligo) or due to the primary destruction of melanocytes, following surgery or cryosurgery. There is no treatment.

Urticaria

Characterized by the presence of round elevations of the skin which may be called 'wheals' or 'plaques'. The initial small lesions may disappear or develop into large plaques and can involve large areas of the body. Urticarial lesions may be present with or without systemic reaction. On occasions pruritus may be present.

Diagnosis is made from the clinical signs but must be differentiated from insect bites and purpura haemorrhagica.

Treatment is frequently not required. In more severe cases, in particular if lung involvement is detected, parenteral administration of antihistamine, corticosteroid and diuretic drugs should be considered. If the horse is seriously ill an adrenergic drug (adrenaline) should be given as soon as possible.

Parasitic dermatoses

External parasitic infection in the horse is typified by extreme irritation, change in disposition and even self-mutilation. The majority of 'itchy' horses have an ectoparasitic problem. The possibility of other causes of pruritus in horses should be considered after eliminating the possibility of the primary cause being an ectoparasite.

Culicoides dermatitis or 'sweet itch'

A seasonal allergic dermatitis affecting all species, irrespective of age, breed or sex.

Clinical signs
The first signs may be seen at any age

Rubbing of tail and mane, in particular, leading to scaling, excoriation, crusting of withers, tail, head and even the whole body in severely affected animals

May get gross thickening of the skin with repeated episodes over the years
Intensity of signs varies with individual horses and worsens with age

Diagnosis
Seasonal clinical signs with response to therapy following elimination of other possible causes.

Differential diagnosis
Ringworm – no itch
Mange
Oxyuris infection
Allergic response to *Stomoxys* bites
Dermatophilus

Treatment
It is better to remove the challenge and allow the signs to subside but this is not always easy

In severely affected cases it may be necessary to provide immediate relief with corticosteroids

Prevention
Once a diagnosis has been made, preventive measures must be instituted and carried on until the end of the *Culicoides* season

For following years, preventive measures must commence prior to the challenge, i.e. at the start of April

House in a stable or box during periods of the day when *Culicoides* are active, possibly with the open door of the box protected with fine mesh material. The stable or box walls can be regularly coated with insecticide, e.g. Stomoxyn P or Rycopel

Following grooming, wipe the horse with a light mineral oil to which an insecticide and/or fly repellent can be added

Use hoods and sheets to provide a physical barrier

Filarial dermatitis

Onchocerca microfilarial larvae are said to congregate in the upper dermis of the head, ventral abdomen and thorax.

Clinical signs
Alopecia, scaling, depigmentation, erythema and crusting.

Diagnosis
History, clinical signs and biopsy.

Treatment
Anthelmintics – fenbendazole and mebendazole at daily doses for five days followed by monthly doses has been suggested.

Fly problems

Fly strike
The flies are attracted to wounds and moist areas, where they lay their eggs. The larvae penetrate living tissue causing extensive damage to the sub-cutaneous tissue and may allow secondary bacterial infection to develop.

Treatment
Clip the area, cleanse the wound, remove the larvae (by flushing the cavity if necessary) with topical application of antibiotic supported by parenteral antibiotic therapy if necessary.

Prevention
Ensure wounds are cleaned and checked regularly for evidence of a 'strike'. Wound dressing used at high risk times should contain insecticidal medications.

Musca infestation
May also be known as 'fly worry'.

Clinical signs

An ulcerative dermatitis, especially of the medial canthus of the eye but may involve the eyelids, nose and lips of the vulva

Irritation and increased lachrymation (this attracts more flies and leads to further fly damage)

Differential diagnosis

Squamous cell carcinoma.

Treatment

Topical application of cream containing an insecticide, e.g. Lorexane

Head hoods of fine mesh material

Simulium

Presents as a pruritic otitis externa with head rubbing and shaking. Crusting may be present in the inner pinna. A non-pruritic form, with white plaques (hyperkeratosis) may also be seen.

Control of Simulium is difficult. Fine mesh hoods, or the use of insecticidal/repellent products may help.

Stable fly

Stomoxys calcitrans cause annoyance to the horse or give painful bites. May also be a vector for blood-borne disease.

Clinical signs

Skin swellings, with intense irritation (stamp feet and swish tail) which may on occasions resemble hypersensitivity reactions

Crust formation may follow where the bite took place

Treatment

None, other than topical antiseptic preparations or antihistamine

If a significant hypersensitivity reaction takes place it may be necessary to sedate any horse that is very upset

Prevention

Regular topical applications of insecticidal or repellent product

Eliminate breeding grounds – decaying moist vegetation and manure heaps (in particular badly kept ones). Insecticidal preparations are available for treating stable walls and areas around dung heaps to reduce the fly population, e.g. Stomoxyn P (Coopers)

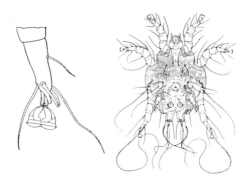

Fig. 7.1 *Chorioptes* sp. Distal end of leg, showing the bell-shaped caruncle (sucker) on its unsegmented stalk.

Mange

Chorioptic mange
The chorioptic mange mite has a 2–3-week life cycle and can live off the host for 2–3 days

Clinical signs
Horse is restless and stamps its feet
Hair loss leading to alopecia
Variable amount of excoriation, exudate and crusting
Lower limbs affected but there can be spread to axilla and inguinal regions and along the ventral chest and abdomen

Diagnosis
Clinical signs and skin scrape – rounded body, short, unjointed pedicles (see Fig. 7.1)

Differential diagnosis
Greasy heel
S. westeri larvae – from wet yards involving the skin around the coronet and pastern

Treatment
Repeated applications of ectoparasiticides, e.g. benzene hexachloride (BHC)

Demodectic mange
Extremely uncommon – localized areas of scaling, hair loss and pustular types have been recorded

Treatment is with ectoparasiticides, particularly Rotenone and organo-phosphates.

Psoroptic mange

Psoroptes equi can live off the host for three weeks and has a two-week life cycle.

Clinical signs

May be only as a pruritic otitis externa – may be presented as a 'head shaker'

Lesions usually start at the base of mane and base of tail but can start on any part of the body that is thickly covered with hair

Alopecia and papules

Self-inflicted trauma leads to erosion and crusting

Scabs remain moist

Diagnosis

Clinical signs with skin scrape – rounded body with long, jointed pedicles

Differential diagnosis

Sarcoptic mange – scabs forming over lesions do not remain moist

Treatment

Ectoparasiticides

Sarcoptic mange

Clinical signs

Intense pruritus with development of small hairless patches on the head, neck, and shoulder, but can affect the whole body

Serum exudes from the lesions to form a dry scab

Diagnosis

Clinical signs with a deep skin scrape – the fourth pair of legs of *Sarcoptes scabiei* do not extend beyond the margin of the body

Treatment

Ectoparasiticides

Oxyuris

A nematode parasite which may give pruritic signs

Clinical signs

Rubbing of tail leads to broken hairs, erosion and even ulcers on tail head and hindquarters.

Diagnosis

Find eggs (clear acetate sticky tape applied to anal and perineal region will remove the eggs, which can be identified microscopically).

N.B. Eggs are not in the faeces – faecal egg counts are not of assistance in diagnosis.

Treatment

Wash perineum and apply vaseline or antiseptic cream
Anthelmintic therapy
Sedatives may be required if there is severe pruritus

Pediculosis – lice

Biting louse – *Haematopinus asini* (see Fig. 7.2a)
Sucking louse – *Damalinia equi* (see Fig. 7.2b)
   A common disease more prevalent in the winter and early spring.

Clinical signs

Dull scaly coat
Pruritus with rubbing and possible self-trauma, affecting the dorsum of the
   body, head, neck and flanks in particular
Severe cases – loss of condition and anaemia

Diagnosis

Physical examination and identification of the parasite and egg cases in the
   coat
The numbers present before rubbing starts varies

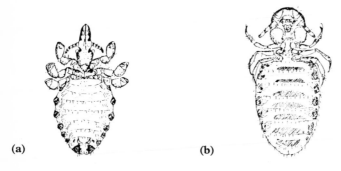

(a)   (b)

Fig. 7.2(a) *Haematopinus asini.* **(b)** *Damalinia equi.*

Treatment
Ectoparasiticides which should be used routinely as a preventive measure.

Warbles

Unable to complete its life cycle in the non-ruminant host. It is advisable to inform the Divisional Veterinary Officer of any cases. The warble fly may annoy the horse.

Clinical signs
Nodules (one or several) which may have a breathing pore on the dorsum, particularly over the withers.

Diagnosis
History, clinical signs with biopsy if necessary – degeneration and necrosis of collagen surrounded by eosinophils and granulomatous infiltration.

Treatment
Poultice or hot fomentation
Excise if necessary
N.B. The use of ectoparasitic drugs may kill the migrating warble, when it may abscessate.

Non-infectious skin dermatoses

Few are important as clinical problems but they must be considered in the differential diagnoses of other diseases.

Nodular skin disease or necrobiosis

Aetiology is unknown but has been thought to be hypersensitivity or microfilarial reactions.

Clinical signs
Nodules appear (not painful) in the dermis of the neck, shoulder and saddle area in particular.

Diagnosis
The presence of non-painful fibrous nodules in these sites is virtually diagnostic but can be confirmed by biopsy – primary change is collagen fibres which have an amorphous, granular appearance.

Treatment
None – may show spontaneous regression. There is no reason why the horse should not be ridden when the fibrous nodules are under the saddle.

Pressure sores

The result of poor management, poorly maintained or ill-fitting saddle or harness, or overtight bandages or support bandages fitted without adequate gamgee or cotton wool. In foals, their very thin, sensitive skin requires very careful padding under bandages, especially over bony prominences.

Treatment
1   Remove cause.
2   Rest from work.
3   Astringent or antibacterial applications.

Burns

Burns are classified by the extent of tissue involvement. Initially there is a diffuse oedema of the skin and subcutaneous tissue, blistering and slough formation.

Treatment
1   Extensive and severe cases must be euthanased.
2   Local damage may require topical dressings to minimize fluid loss and infection. The use of 'Flamazine' cream (Smith and Nephew) will assist in the control of *Pseudomonas* species.

Photosensitization

1   Primary (direct) – erythema, oedema and necrosis by ultraviolet light on the skin, particularly the white areas. The treatment is by removal from sunlight and, if necessary, corticosteroid and anti-histamine creams can be used.
2   Secondary (indirect) – depends on the degree of liver dysfunction and has a poor prognosis.

Dry coat

Found in horses introduced to the tropics from temperate climates without a period of acclimatization. It is considered an exhaustion of the sweating mechanisms, giving a dry scurfy skin. The horse recovers if removed to a temperate climate.

Grease, greasy heel

Seen predominantly in the heavy horse or horses with a lot of 'feather' on the legs. It is recognized as a complication of a primary dermatitis, frequently parasitic in origin, e.g. *Chorioptes equi*.

Treatment is by clipping out lower limb, cleansing and, if appropriate, applying ectoparasitic treatment.

Hyperelastica cutis

A condition similar to Ehlers–Danlos syndrome with the excessive production of fragile skin and abnormal collagen. Surgical removal of the excessive skin has been reported but is unlikely to be successful as multifocal areas of the trunk are involved.

Common neoplasias

Melanoma
Commonly affect grey and dappled grey horses over six years of age
Multiple lesions around the anus, vulva, prepuce, in the abdomen, subcutaneous tissues over the body. May become malignant
Surgical treatment is difficult and ultimately unlikely to be successful

Neurofibroma
Small, firm, nodular lesions within the skin of the eyelids and must be differentiated from sarcoids
Remove surgically

Squamous cell carcinoma
Clinically appear as an ulcerated area of granulation tissue commonly on the nose, lips, nictating membrane, conjunctiva and genitalia
Treatment is by surgical removal

Bacterial dermatoses

Abscess
Frequently associated with puncture wounds or a tooth abscess
Treatment is by poultice or hot fomentations until the abscess ruptures or, when considered necessary, incision and drainage
An abscess which has ruptured spontaneously may also need an incision at its lowest dependent point. There follows cleansing of the cavity and surrounding area of skin
See also 'Bacterial folliculitis and furunculosis (acne)', below

Bacterial folliculitis and furunculosis (acne)

Folliculitis, due to bacteria or fungi, is inflammation of the hair follicles. When there is spread to the surrounding dermis and subcutis it is called furunculosis. If these areas coalesce, a boil or abscess is formed.

Lesions frequently occur under the saddle or places in contact with harness and are associated with poor grooming, dirty tack and badly managed stables. Abscesses may also occur at the commissures of the mouth. The lesions may be single but are usually multiple. Swabs may be taken to identify the causal organisms, commonly staphylococci but others such as *Corynebacterium* species may be found.

Treatment is initially to improve stable hygiene. Wash all tack and grooming kit in antiseptic solution (chlorhexidine or iodophor products). Wash all lesions daily with an antiseptic shampoo, and discard or boilwash any cloths after each use.

In some cases parenteral and topical antibiotics are necessary. Autogenous vaccines have been used with variable results.

Dermatophilus

May be called 'rain scald', 'mud fever', etc. Caused by *Dermatophilus congolensis* and characterized by exudation, scab formation and loss of hair. There may be a secondary bacterial infection, e.g. staphylococci.

Clinical signs
Vary with the length of coat – long-haired horses have more hair matting and larger scab formation. Removal of the scab shows a moist, pink skin, which may be raised slightly and have an ovoid shape. In short-haired horses the scabs are smaller with the hairs embedded in the scab, which is easily pulled free from the skin with fingers.

Around the fetlock, pastern and bulbs of the heels there is an initial exudate, scab formation and matting of the hair. This can be followed by oedema, cracking with further exudation and oedema, and lameness.

Diagnosis
Demonstration of *D. congolensis* from fresh lesions in stained smear or following culture on blood agar. The demonstration of the organism in old or healing lesions is more difficult. Microscopic examination of smears stained with methylene blue will show the presence of branching, mycelium-forming organisms. Giemsa stain and squash preparation can also be used.

Treatment
Keep the horse dry – no contact with wet, muddy fields and keep out of the
    rain

Remove the debris and, where suitable, the scabs, using a disinfectant shampoo, e.g. surgical scrub preparations, and apply a 1% potash of alum solution or allow the skin to dry out

When necessary, parenteral antibiotics should be given – procaine penicillin is a drug of choice (a penicillin/streptomycin combination may also be used)

Prevention or control

Prolonged wet weather exacerbates the condition, in particular in horses kept in muddy fields with no opportunity for the mud on the limbs and body to dry out (or be removed)

If possible, stable the horse in a dry box. If the horse is 'prone' to mud fever, ensure the bedding is kept dry or remove the bedding for most of the day

Ensure regular, good grooming (with cleaning of grooming kit and prompt attention to any skin lesions)

Ulcerative lymphangitis

See Chapter 11.

Viral dermatoses

Coital exanthema

A venereal disease of horses including the penis and prepuce of the male, the vulva and perineum of the mare. The causal agent is the equine herpes virus, EHV-3.

Clinical signs

Watery blisters initially which progress to circumscribed areas with yellow necrotic tops

Occasional oedema of the prepuce

Vulva oedematous within hours of the blisters appearing, 4–7 days after service by an infected stallion

Diagnosis

Provisional diagnosis from clinical signs confirmed by virus isolation (in vesicular stage) or paired samples at one month interval for serum neutralization and complement fixation tests.

Differential diagnosis

Bacterial infection.

Treatment

Cessation of service until regression and healing of lesions

Washing with 1:100 chlorhexidine for 3–5 days
Antibiotic or chlorhexidine cream applied daily

Papillomatosis

A highly infectious viral skin disease of horses up to 3–4 years of age.

Clinical signs
Short-stalked, warty growths on muzzle, nose, eyelids and occasionally on
    the neck and forelimbs
All in-contact young horses are affected
Variable number of the growths present which are larger if only two or three
    are present
As the warts mature over 3–4 months there is a change from grey to pinkish
    colour

Diagnosis
Clinical appearance, distribution and age of animal with a biopsy for
histopathology if uncertain.

Differential diagnosis
Sarcoid – may be very similar to the larger warts
Fibroma

Treatment
None, as the majority slough in 3-4 weeks of reaching maturity but various
    therapies have been advocated – cryosurgery, chemical cautery
Vaccination, with a formalin treated suspension of warts from affected
    horses, has been suggested but is probably of more relevance in the
    treatment of cases where the warts are persistently active
Treatment will be necessary if there is fly strike and secondary infection

Prevention
Paddock fences and stables should be thoroughly cleansed and disinfected
by a chemical that kills the virus, e.g. formaldehyde.

Congenital papilloma in foals
Black wart-like growths on the skin of newborn foals
They are treated by application of a ligature, or where there is a wide base, by
    surgical removal under local analgesia

Sarcoid

A common cutaneous tumour with no predilection for age, breed, sex or
colour.

Clinical signs

There are two clinical entities:

Verrucous type – slow growing, either sessile or pedunculated and characteristically dry, horny and cauliflower-like in appearance.

Fibroblastic type – start as hard fibrous nodules which are grey/white to yellow on section. They increase in size and erode through the epidermis, become traumatized and rapidly have a proud flesh appearance.

In addition, there are the **mixed types**, where both verrucous and fibroblastic type sarcoid are present and **nodular alopecia** which is characterized by a hairless area with one or two dermal nodules. The nodular alopecia type may remain dormant for many years and regress spontaneously, but on injury (or surgery) it will develop a significant fibroblastic reaction.

Diagnosis

Can be difficult as they resemble many other conditions

Complete removal is preferred to biopsy as incomplete removal will produce a significant fibroblastic reaction

Treatment

Ligature – pedunculated sarcoids

Surgical removal – disappointing results with regrowth in up to 50% of cases. Surgical removal may be necessary where it is unsuitable to use cryosurgery, e.g. over the eye

Cryosurgery – produces the most consistent results

Vaccination or stimulation of the immune system – BCG vaccine

Radiation therapy – must be done by a qualified radiologist

Prognosis

Always give a guarded prognosis

The prognosis for a horse which has had previous unsuccessful treatment is less favourable

Dermatomycosis

The most prevalent causative organisms are *Trichophyton* (*T. equinum* is by far the most common but *T. mentagrophytes* and *verrucosum* are associated with infection) and *Microsporum*.

Natural infection is by direct contact with infected animals and indirect transmission by brushes, tack, stable woodwork, etc.

Clinical signs

Trichophytosis

Incubation period 5–10 days following contact

Hair loss at 3–10 days

T. equinum – small rounded patches which gradually enlarge

Vesicles form in the hairless area, rupture and form scabs

Irritation present at this time

T. mentagrophytes – most lesions on the head, neck and base of tail as rounded or irregular lesions of varying sizes with greyish crusts

T. verrucosum – seen commonly in horses that grazed with, or had access to buildings which housed ringworm-infected cattle. Lesions similar to above with some local irritation

Microsporum sp. – small round lesions with scales – with *M. gyseum* infection the lesions will be larger and more inflamed. On removal of the crusts there is a moist, reddish ulcer

Diagnosis

The clinical signs are frequently very suggestive of ringworm but confirmation can be obtained by examination of skin scrape or culture of sample.

Aids to diagnosis

Skin scrape

Culture – dermatophyte medium or Sabouraud's medium

Wood's lamp – possible fluorescence *M. equinum* and *M. canis* not *Trichophyton* sp.

Treatment

Topical fungicides which can also be used on grooming kit and tack

Oral griseofulvin has been used but is of questionable efficiency as the drug may not be incorporated into infected hair. Should use topical fungicides concurrently with griseofulvin

N.B. Do not use griseofulvin in pregnant mares.

8 / Diseases of the musculoskeletal system

Exertional rhabdomyolysis

Azoturia – the name for the severe form of the disease
Monday morning disease – the disease occurs after the horse has been
   rested for a day or more, which in the working horse is after the weekend
Tying up – appears to represent a milder form of the disease
Cases can be seen at any stage during an exercise period. It is frequently seen
   when training is interrupted by weather, injury or management
   difficulties or in endurance horses after extreme exertion

Clinical signs

Mild cases
Stiffness (perhaps transient)
Gait abnormalities
No discoloration of the urine

Severe cases
Reluctant or unable to move
Muscle stiffness with pain and tremors, or spasms, in particular in the
   muscles of the back and hindquarters
Elevated pulse and respiratory rates
Urine may be reddish-brown to almost black depending on the amount of
   myoglobin present

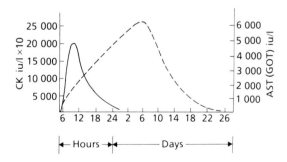

Fig. 8.1 Pattern of enzyme levels in sequential blood samples after clinical signs of
exertional rhabdomyolysis.

Diagnosis
From history and presenting clinical signs
Laboratory confirmation may be essential depending on the severity and
clinical signs present

Diagnostic aids
Blood chemistry – CK (creatinine kinase) and AST (aspartate amino-
transferase) are normally used (see Fig. 8.1)
CK values rise rapidly in the course of the disease and drop rapidly to half
value over the next 12 hours and are almost back to normal by 24 hours.
Elevation greater than 188 iu/litre and possibly thousands. Continuing
elevation of CK values indicate ongoing damage
AST rises more slowly and takes 10–12 days to return to normal
Sequential samples should be taken, in particular with the milder forms of
the disease, to evaluate the degree of muscle damage accurately. In
milder forms, a sample before exercise, one 10 minutes after exercise,
followed by one 24 hours later should be considered the minimum
necessary to give an accurate diagnosis
Urine analysis – reagent 'dip sticks' may be used to detect the presence of
myoglobin and haemoglobin
Visible changes in colour if myoglobin exceeds 40 mg/ml – warn owners

Treatment
Administer a non-steroidal anti-inflammatory drug (NSAID), e.g. phe-
nylbutazone or flunixin
Fluids and electrolytes in severe cases – use a balanced electrolyte solution
with a bicarbonate precursor, e.g. lactated Ringer's solution intrave-
nously. Oral electrolyte can be used later
Larger doses of corticosteroids, e.g. 40–60 mg betamethasone, intrave-
nously counteracts shock and stabilizes cellular membranes
Vitamin B, vitamin E and selenium may assist in the recovery phase
Walking exercise
High fibre diet

Prognosis
Recovery should be monitored by serial serum enzyme levels. This should
determine when it is suitable to return the horse from limited walking to
exercise and may take 2–3 weeks.
    The return to work should be at a lower rate than previously and must
not be too soon. Horses which suffer repeated episodes are often not suitable
for the purpose for which they are kept.
    The prognosis is better if the carbohydrate intake is kept as low as is
compatible with conditions and satisfactory performance. An opportunity

should be taken to look at the horse's normal diet. Dietary supplementation with vitamin E and selenium has been suggested for prophylaxis.

Nutritional myopathy

Seen in foals but possible also in adults.

Oral supplement of 1.5–4.4 mg/kg bodyweight of vitamin E per day. Selenium supplements will not replace the need for vitamin E supplementation if vitamin E is deficient. See also Chapter 13.

Acute myopathy

Has been reported in horses at grass in east and south-east Scotland and resembles clinical signs of paralytic myoglobinuria. Passage of dark brown urine and grossly increased creatine kinase activities were consistent but selenium status varied from normal to deficient. The muscles of posture and respiration rather than movement were affected. Most of the affected horses died.

Exhaustion

Clinical signs
Heart and respiratory rate above 60 per minute for more than 15 minutes after exercise has ceased
Pyrexia 103–107°F
Cardiac arrhythmias
Muscle twitching and fasciculations
Dehydration – profound
Depression – possible disorientation

Treatment
Cooling may be necessary
NSAIDs
Fluid therapy – 20 to 40 litres i.v.
Bicarbonate contraindicated

'Stopping'

Complete depletion of muscle glycogen and free fatty acids (FFA). Horse comes to a complete halt and is incapable of moving, yet is bright and alert. Able to move, unaided, in less than one hour.

Hypocalcaemia (See also Chapter 13)

Relatively rare disorder of lactating mares or following hard work or transport.

Clinical signs
Variable, including:
    stiff stilted gait
    muscle fasciculations
    ataxia
    anxiety
    sweating
    elevated body temperature
    convulsions, coma and death

Diagnosis
Clinical signs with history of lactation, transport or prolonged exercise
    suggestive
Confirm with blood sample if values below 6 mg/dl

Differential diagnosis
Tetanus

Treatment
Mild cases may recover spontaneously but therapy recommended. Calcium borogluconate at 250–500 ml/500 kg diluted 1:4 with saline or dextrose.

Malignant oedema

The causal organism is usually *Clostridium septicum*, with *perfringens* and *chauvoei* also possible, which may gain entry to the body through cuts, wounds, surgical interference and contaminated needles.

Clinical signs
Signs appear 12–45 hours after inoculation

Early signs
Soft pitting oedema
Little gas formation
Lesions spread rapidly

Later signs
Pain over affected area with crepitus

Infiltration with large quantities of gelatinous exudate and emphysema. May
  ooze sero-sanguinous fluid
Fever
Anorexia and depression
Lameness if a limb is involved
Signs of toxaemia develop

Post-mortem findings
Dark haemorrhagic muscle
Extensive subcutaneous oedema

Diagnosis
From clinical signs, especially if there is a history of local injury. Can be
supported by Gram stain of exudate.

Differential diagnosis
Azoturia
Colic

Treatment
Parenteral antibiotics – penicillin specifically, 50 000 iu/kg i.v.
Fluid therapy if shock or toxaemia present
Surgical drainage of the oedematous site and introduction of oxygen
Analgesics
Non-steroidal anti-inflammatory drugs

Prognosis
Unless antibiotic therapy is instituted very early, the disease is usually fatal
within 1–4 days from the onset of symptoms.

Sporadic lymphangitis

A painful non-contagious disease of a hind leg, usually occurring in horses
fed a highly nutritious ration with restricted exercise for a few days. The
aetiology is unknown but is usually associated with superficial wounds to the
lower limb and is thought to develop as a lymphangitis.

Clinical signs
Limb is hot and swollen
Severe pain – the horse may refuse to put its foot to the ground
Systemic reaction – fever, sweating anorexia, elevated pulse and respiration
Swelling may extend to the inguinal region with involvement of the regional
  lymph nodes

Diagnosis

From the clinical signs and history. It is not unusual for cases to be seen if there is a sudden prolonged period of icing on yards and roads preventing horses from leaving their boxes, especially if owners do not immediately cut the ration.

Treatment

Parenteral antibiotics – penicillin or other antibiotic

Phenylbutazone to produce analgesia and allow the horse to move

Diuretic – e.g. Lasix and a laxative

Hot fomentations, upward massage of the limb followed by bandaging (with ample cotton wool padding) to minimize swelling and decrease the risk of protein exudation through the skin

Gentle exercise

Prognosis

Most cases improve within a few days once gentle exercise is started

Some permanent thickening of the limb may occur

Recurrences are common in the same limb

Prevention

Prompt and careful treatment of all wounds of the lower limb

Decrease the animal's feed in proportion to the amount of work done. If the horse has been on a high level of nutrition it may be beneficial to give a bran mash following the sudden reduction in feed

9 / Cardiovascular system

Examination of the cardiovascular system may be carried out for a variety of reasons. This can be in conjunction with a sale or a proposal for insurance, on finding suspicious signs during a clinical examination or following a report of poor performance.

The heart and the peripheral system have a close and dynamic interaction and must not be considered as two components.

Disease of the heart can reflect, or have profound effects on, systemic health, as can lesions affecting local perfusion affect the heart and circulation. The cardiovascular system has considerable reserves and will compensate for disease in most cases by circulatory haemostatic mechanisms.

A good clinical approach to the system requires a thorough general examination of the horse at rest and an assessment of response to exercise. This includes inspection of the mucosa, determining the rate, rhythm and character of the arterial pulse, auscultation of the heart and lungs, percussion of the thorax and looking for evidence of a jugular pulse, excessive sweating and oedema.

Clinical examination

General
Observe general attitude and appearance

Assess colour of all visible mucous membranes and capillary refill time

Look for evidence of oedema, in particular ventral oedema

Establish the arterial pulse which is obtained by palpating a peripheral artery
and examining for rate, rhythm and character. Irregularities present at
rest, which disappear on exercise, are not uncommon

The resting rate should be 30 to 40 beats per minute (25–45) but is greatly
influenced by the horse's temperament

An increased resting heart rate (>50 beats/minute) may be associated with:
- febrile conditions
- painful conditions
- cardiac disease
- anaemia (haemorrhage)

The character of the arterial pulse is full and strong in a normal horse.
Alterations may be from:
- arrhythmias
- cardiac lesions of left side of heart

- mitral incompetence or stenosis – weak pulse
- aortic incompetence – shortened pulse
N.B. Precordial thrill is always abnormal

Observe jugular pulse, which most horses show at the thoracic inlet, due to pulsations of the underlying carotid artery. If the head is erect it is normal to see slight movement for up to 10 cm above the thoracic inlet

Ensure both jugular veins are patent:
>   Distension without pulsation:
>   thrombosis
>   cranial vena cava obstruction
>   mediastinal neoplasia
>   Distension with pulse:
>   right-sided heart failure
>   tricuspid valve regurgitation
>   atrial fibrillation

Auscultate both lungs and heart. The arterial pulse should be palpated while the heart is being auscultated

>   N.B. Many of the signs result from other than cardiac disease e.g. respiratory crackles, dyspnoea and exercise intolerance is most likely to indicate a respiratory problem.

Where there is a problem with the circulation, the following may be found:
>   Interference with arterial supply:
>   loss of pulse
>   coldness
>   blanching of tissues
>   pain/spasm
>   Interference with venous drainage:
>   distended veins
>   swelling
>   oedema
>   cyanosis, distal to lesion
>   Interference with capillaries:
>   extravasion of fluid
>   reddening
>   petechial haemorrhages

Intravenous injections and catheters

Inflammation of the vein wall and thrombophlebitis is not uncommon following injection of drugs which are chemically irritant, e.g. phenylbutazone, inadvertent perivascular injection or prolonged use of intravenous catheters. The relatively few reports in veterinary literature suggest the incidence and types of organisms isolated are similar to those reported in the medical literature. The most commonly isolated organisms were *Staphylococcus* spp., *Corynebacterium* spp., *Enterobacter* spp. and *Streptococcus* spp., with horses with severe disease and foals more prone to develop complications of the catheter site. It is uncertain if colonization is at the time of insertion or during use. Removal of peripheral catheters between 48 and 72 hours is now widely practised in human medicine.

Intravenous catheterization provides a direct line to the circulatory system. Insertion should be only with stringent aseptic techniques, e.g. using iodine or chlorhexidine, and proper subsequent management, such as the application of antiseptics around the insertion site, is essential. Use of catheters with smooth topography discourages thrombus deposition, microbial adherence and subsequent colonization, while use of a scalpel facilitates insertion and reduces local damage.

Insertion site infections which are uncomplicated usually respond to antibiotics, as do catheter-related septicaemias, whereas those with complications such as a septic thrombus may not.

The risk of thrombus formation is greatly reduced if catheters and needles of smooth topography are used.

Examination of the heart

The heart should be examined, in a quiet site, at rest and at exercise in relation to the degree of fitness. Each horse will be presented with a different level of fitness and must be treated individually.

The exercise part should follow a standard protocol and increase in severity, with assessment by auscultation and of the pulse, immediately after each period of work. The examination should stop if there are findings which suggest any possible risk to the rider, or to the horse, by further exercise.

Start with the horse at rest

Followed by trot up in hand

Then lunge and or ride – the initial ridden period should be some two minutes. Ridden exercise is preferable, if possible, to lunge for the 'strenuous exercise' part of the examination

Auscultation should continue for several minutes as the heart slows. The longer the period of exercise, the greater the time to regain the resting rate. In addition to assessing return of heart rate to normal after exercise, the mucous membrane colour and distension of the jugular vein should also be assessed.

Heart sounds

The valve areas are heard:
• Tricuspid: at the 3rd or 4th intercostal space

- Mitral: at the 5th left intercostal space
- Aortic: anterior border of 4th left rib on level of shoulder joint
- Pulmonic: at the 3rd left intercostal space below the shoulder joint

Murmurs

Although murmurs may be associated with heart disease they are often not relevant and may not be associated with lesions at post-mortem. 'Innocent murmurs' are found in more than 50% of horses with a functional murmur between sound one and sound two reported in 20% of fit horses.

Cardiac murmurs mean less during the newborn period than at any other time in the horse's life.

With a patent ductus arteriosus there is a continuous sound which decreases with age and often is not heard for more than the first two days of life.

Classification of murmurs
Grade 1: requires absolute quiet and concentration
Grade 2: soft and localised to one area
Grade 3: immediately audible when stethoscope placed over cardiac area
Grade 4: loud and audible over most of the chest but not audible unless stethoscope is in contact with the skin
Grade 5: heard without stethoscope contact with the skin

Soft, Grade 2 or less murmurs during systole or diastole without other signs are probably benign. Functional murmurs, not associated with heart disease, are most easily heard over the heart base.

Systolic murmurs, of low intensity, begin in early systole and end before second heart sound, commonly originate from the aortic/pulmonary valves.

Murmurs of Grade 3 or more should be regarded as significant.

Atrioventricular murmurs – systolic is usually holosystolic with regurgitation usually heard over the mitral valve area. Common causes are degenerative valve disease and bacterial endocarditis. Diastolic murmurs are rare.

A murmur occupying the whole systolic period or a murmur accompanied by a palpable thrill reflects cardiac disease. Gross murmurs require investigation using ECG and possibly, if available, echocardiography. Significant murmurs may become so faint as to be inaudible in the presence of atrial fibrillation. The murmur may reappear if sinus rhythm is restored.

Congenital heart disease

Not very common in horses. Most frequently reported are ventricular septal defects and patent ductus arteriosus. Multiple cardiac anomalies, such as tetralogy of Fallot and Eisenmenger's complex have been reported.

Very serious heart anomalies may not be accompanied by any murmur.

Patent ductus arteriosus (PDA)

A closing ductus arteriosus may cause a very loud murmur which is a continuous 'machinery-type' murmur which disappears by 48–96 hours of age. PDA can occur as a single defect or with other anomalies.

Clinical signs
Depend on the size of PDA – large ones produce less, if any, murmur
More severe PDA increases the possibility of congestive heart failure
Direct visualization of the PDA with echocardiography is difficult in neonates

Treatment
The condition can be corrected surgically in neonates.

Prognosis
Poor if large defect
Horse may have small defect through life with no symptoms

Ventricular septal defects (VSD)

An opening in the septum between the ventricles, either as a single entity or as part of a complex. They are commonly located in the membranous portion of the septum, ventral to the right coronary cusp of the aortic valve and the septal leaflet of the tricuspid valve.

Clinical signs
Clinical signs vary and depend on the size of defect and whether associated with other defect(s) of heart and/or other organs
When there is a small defect, most horses grow normally and only a murmur is heard
With larger defects, a holosystolic, 'harsh' murmur heard on both sides with a palpable thrill is found
The horse may show poor growth rate, lethargy or exercise intolerance
Dyspnoea, jugular pulse, ventral oedema may be present
When there is cardiac enlargement, or failure, cardiac dysrhythmias may be present

Diagnosis
Suspect a VSD when a holosystolic murmur, with palpable thrill, can be

heard on both sides of the heart. Confirmation is possible with echo-cardiographic examination.

Prognosis
Horses with small defects may be otherwise apparently normal
Intensity of murmur is not a good guide to size of defect
Do not breed from horses with VSD

Arrhythmias

Arrhythmias are identified by the occurrence of variation in the interval between beats, discrepancies between heart and pulse rate, variations in interval between beats, variations in intensity of sounds.

Rhythm disturbances, without detectable heart disease, may be found in horses with toxaemia, septicaemia, anaemia, metabolic disorders and disease of the hepatic, renal or endocrine systems. Use of drugs, e.g. detomidine, xylazine, romifidine, also causes rhythm disturbances.

Arrhythmias occurring in the horse which can be considered to be non-pathogenic include:
- sinus arrhythmia
- wandering pacemaker
- sinoatrial block
- incomplete atrioventricular block with dropped beats

Signs which indicate heart disease include:
- atrial fibrillation
- ventricular extrasystole
- paroxysmal ventricular tachycardia
- complete heart block

Sinus arrythmia

Unusual in the horse
Present at rest, disappears on exercise
No missed beats but readily recognized in an ECG
No clinical significance

Wandering pacemaker

Where the pacemaker function is moving from one part of the heart to another. The locus can move quite long distances and, in the horse, still be within the sino-atrial node. If the pacemaker moves outside the sino-atrial node it is considered a pathological lesion exists
Irregular, possibly cyclical, heart rhythm

Recognized on ECG by changes in form of the P-wave
Benign wandering pacemaker will disappear on light exercise

Sino-atrial block

There is the occasional heartbeat skipped when the pacemaker fails to
initiate a beat, or the beat may be missed in a rhythmic manner, e.g. every
third or fourth beat missing. The following pulse after the missing beat may
be stronger from the increased stroke volume.

Usually associated with slow heart rates with the heart becoming regular
on increased cardiac output.

A horse showing sino-atrial block at exercise must be regarded with some
concern.

Atrioventricular block

Depolarization begins normally in the sino-atrial node and spreads over the
atrial myocardium but its conduction through the atrio-ventricular node is
either delayed or blocked completely. The three common types are described as first, second and third degree atrio-ventricular block. They can be
identified with some accuracy by auscultation and observation but are best
diagnosed electrocardiographically.

First degree block
Prolonged P-Q interval as atrioventricular conduction is delayed. Increased
time between atrial sound and first heart sound with abnormal prominence
of the atrial sound.

Significance is unknown but performance may be reduced.

Second degree block
Commonest cause of loss of normal heart rhythm. All but a few beats are
conducted normally. The atrium depolarizes but the ventricles do not
respond to depolarization at the atrioventricular node, so no QRS complex
or T-wave is seen on ECG.

On auscultation, a first atrial sound with greater than normal engorge-
ment of the jugular vein during the blocked beats. Dropped beats are usually
in a regular pattern and not associated with other findings.

Significance is unknown but probably insignificant if no more than one
beat is dropped and normal rhythm is resumed after light exercise.

If this block is manifest by or continues after excitement or exercise, it
should be considered abnormal. May also be seen immediately after cessation of exercise as the heart slows when there is, transiently, a bizarre
rhythm.

Third degree block

Rare and may be transient. Third degree, or 'complete' block results from isolation of the ventricles from the depolarizing influence of the atria.

Clinical signs include lethargy, slow, regular ventricular rate, engorged jugular veins with 'cannon waves' or 'giant a-waves' and variation in the first heart sound intensity. Diagnosis can be confirmed by ECG.

Important because of the possibility of Adam–Stokes attacks and consequent syncope. The horse is therefore unsafe to ride.

Atrial fibrillation

Sudden loss in performance and stamina usually following strenuous exercise
May disappear within 24 hours
Heart rhythm is chaotic with beats occurring at irregular intervals which may
   be up to 10–12 seconds
Pulse irregular in rhythm and volume
First heart sound very clear – no preceding atrial sound

Diagnosis

Diagnosis can be confirmed from the irregular QRS-complexes and absence of P-waves on ECG. Small, irregular fibrillation waves are also present with the ventricular rate very fast (>120 beats per minute).

Treatment

Quinidine sulphate orally by stomach tube at 10 g (some clinicians give 20 g)
   every 2 hours until sinus rhythm is established or 80g has been given
A test dose of 10 g should be given the previous day

N.B. Side effects are possible which include swelling of nasal mucosa, urticarial wheals, gastrointestinal disturbance, laminitis, cardiovascular collapse, atrioventricular block or sudden death.

Prognosis

Prognosis is better if the atriofibrillation is recent
Poor if concurrent signs of heart murmur or heart failure
A murmur may reappear on restoration of sinus rhythm

Pericardium

Pericarditis

Uncommon in horses but, when present, tends to be fibrinous.

Clinical signs
Muffled heart sounds

Tachycardia

Absence of heart sounds in ventral thorax

Jugular vein distension

Peripheral oedema and cyanotic mucous membranes may be present

Haematological changes not specific but white cell count may be increased
or normal depending on cause

ECG changes most commonly associated with pericarditis are decreased
amplitude of QRS-complexes and S-T elevation or slurring, but in some
animals no changes are evident

Echocardiography can assist in confirming the diagnosis

Treatment
Unrewarding

Antibiotics parenterally can be tried with a very guarded prognosis

Pericardiocentesis with or without lavage and local infusion of antibiotics
has been reported

Prognosis
Very poor and hopeless if signs of congestive heart failure

Endocardium

Vascular disorders

Disorders of the valves are usually acquired. They may be the result of
degenerative changes, infection, inflammation or trauma. Age related
changes, such as nodules or fibrosis, may be present with no apparent effect.

Degenerative changes may lead to aortic insufficiency. Rupture of
chordae tendinae of the mitral valve will lead to acute respiratory distress,
pansystolic murmur and possibly a loud third heart sound. If fever and
murmur both present always consider bacterial endocarditis. Bacterial
endocarditis has a possible association with phlebitis and perivascular
abscessation. Pyogenic infection with valvular endocarditis is not common
but, if present, the right AV valve (tricuspid) is usually affected.

Most reports are of streptococci and *Actinobacillus equuli* present, with
Erysipelothrix rhusiopathiae, Escherichia coli and *Pseudomonas aeruginosa* also
isolated from cases.

Bacterial endocarditis

Bacterial endocarditis can have a varied history and many clinical signs
including:
- Fever

- Oedema of the extremities
- Tachycardia
- Murmurs (loudest on left side and mostly systolic)
- Neutrophilia
- Slight to moderate hyperglobulinaemia

Treatment
Initial treatment with antibiotics effective against Gram +ve and Gram –ve
  organisms
Blood samples for bacterial culture must be taken before treatment is
  instituted. Drug forms that provide rapid maximum therapeutic blood
  levels and penetrate tissue are indicated, e.g. crystalline penicillin salts
  with potentiated sulphonamide trimethoprim combinations

Prognosis
Very poor
Any treatment must be aggressive and intensive to have any chance of success

Myocardial disease

Myocarditis

Inflammation of the myocardial wall of bacterial, viral or parasitic origin. It
may also follow thromboembolic disease. Known bacterial causes include
Streptococcus equi, Staphylococcus aureus and *Clostridium chauvoei.* Viruses
include equine influenza, equine viral arteritis and equine infectious anaemia. Infection with the spirochaete *Borrelia burgdorferi* may be a cause of
myocarditis.

At least 10% of horses have myocardial fibrosis at post-mortem which
has been linked to ischaemia from emboli due to migrating parasitic larvae.
These lesions are probably of no clinical significance.

Clinical signs
Signs are highly variable and may be missed due to predominance of the
  other clinical signs of systemic illness
Usually febrile
Tachycardia – possible sinus tachycardia
Dysrhythmia may be present
Murmur from tricuspid or mitral valve insufficiency
Horse may be unwilling to move or just show exercise intolerance
Jugular vein pulsation and/or distension and signs of congestive heart failure
  may be present

Differential diagnosis

May be difficult to differentiate from septicaemia, respiratory disease and colic or other cardiac disease

Haematology – neutrophilia may not always be present

Blood chemistry – while AST, CK and LDH may be elevated, there may be a contribution from skeletal muscle and liver. The use of specific myocardial isoenzymes is indicated, but care with interpretation as specificity and sensitivity of these tests have not been fully documented in large animals

Non-specific inflammation

This may be associated with infection, e.g. respiratory tract virus or strangles, and may well follow a horse being exercised in the early stages of the disease.

Stop exercise immediately and turn horse away for 2–3 months.

Toxic degeneration

Most common reported cause is ionophore, monensin or salinomycin poisoning. In addition to myocardial damage, skeletal muscle, hepatic and renal disturbances are also present. See Chapter 12.

Specific cardiovascular findings reported include:

- Paroxysmal atrial tachycardia/multiple ventricular extrasystoles
- Dull, muffled heart sound – pericardial and pleural effusions
- Jugular pulse with marked depression of S-T segment on ECG
- Atrial fibrillation – which does not respond to quinidine.

10/Neurological disease

For most of the conditions there is no specific treatment and supportive or symptomatic therapies frequently produce little or no significant improvement.

Cerebellar disease

Cerebellar hypoplasia has been reported in Arabian foals. The clinical signs may be present following birth or appear within the first months of age.

Clinical signs
Intention tremor
Ataxia – mild incoordination to inability to stand
Reduced blink reflex

Cerebral disease

May be unilateral or bilateral involvement with very variable clinical signs. The causes include:

Unilateral disease
Focal abscess (*S. equi*)
Focal protozoan encephalitis
Aberrant strongyle larvae

Bilateral disease
Aberrant strongyle larvae
Eastern equine encephalitis (EEE), Western equine encephalitis (WEE), Venezuelan equine encephalitis (VEE), rabies
Hepatic encephalopathy

Clinical signs
From depression, disorientation through to hyperexcitability and aggressive behaviour
Aimless wandering
Head pressing
Circling
    If ataxia or paresis is present there is brain stem or spinal cord involvement.

Spinal cord disease

Trauma
From vertebral fractures, epiphyseal separations (especially in foals) and luxation at atlas and axis (especially in foals which have 'gone over' backwards).

Clinical signs
Ataxia
Weakness
Spasticity
All four limbs affected with cervical injury, pelvic limbs only with an injury between T2 and S2 vertebrae.

Diagnosis
The clinical findings can be supported by radiographical examination. This is restricted to the neck using portable X-ray machine. It is frequently difficult to keep the animal still to get radiographs in the two planes necessary and the resulting plates may be very difficult to interpret.

Treatment
Corticosteroids, as soon as possible following the injury. Initial dose 4 mg betamethasone/50 kg bodyweight i.v. Further doses of 2 mg/50 kg bodyweight should be given daily for a further three days. Surgical treatment is unlikely to be practical in most cases.

Cervical vertebral stenotic myelopathy

A focal compressive lesion of the cervical spinal cord due to a narrowed spinal canal. They are frequently referred to as 'wobblers', but this term refers to a syndrome and does not imply any one particular cause of the syndrome. The stenosis is usually found at C3 or C4 but can be from C1 to C7 vertebrae.

Clinical signs
Young animals (6–12 months) predominate
Ataxia, weakness and spasticity appear in the pelvic limbs first
Acute onset of signs with variable progression
Highest incidence is in thoroughbreds, but can be seen in any breed

Diagnosis
The presence of clinical signs in an old foal or yearling thoroughbred.
Radiographic examination may assist – lateral view. It may be necessary to use contrast medium in some cases but this procedure is not without

some risk to the patient. It requires general anaesthesia and may be considered as a final confirmatory procedure prior to euthanasia if the owner required such confirmation.

Vertebral osteomyelitis

Due to bacteria, e.g. *Mycobacterium, Brucella, Corynebacterium* species, and is seen more frequently in foals or young horses as a sequel to a septicaemia.

Clinical findings
Signs of pressure on the spinal cord. The findings depend on the level at which the lesion occurs. The clinical signs are sudden in onset, progressive and need not be found during the period of septicaemia.

Diagnosis
The clinical findings are usually very suggestive but radiography and haematology may assist.

Treatment
Usually unrewarding. In the early stages, antibacterial therapy in high doses with drainage (if possible).

Equine degenerative myeloencephalopathy

A diffuse degenerative disease of the spinal cord and brain. It is possibly of toxic, nutritional or metabolic aetiology.

Clinical signs
Symmetrical ataxia
Most frequently seen in the 6-month to 2-year-old horse

Diagnosis
The diagnosis requires careful neurological examination. The degrees of gait deficit are more consistent with a diffuse spinal cord disease than a focal lesion (e.g. as in vertebral osteomyelitis above).

Treatment
No therapy is suggested
Supportive therapy may be required until a diagnosis is made

Equine motor neurone disease

Confirmed cases have been reported in North America with, in early 1993, a report of possible cases in the United Kingdom. Defined as a motor neurone disease confined almost exclusively to changes in the lower motor neurones in the ventral horn of the spinal cord.

Clinical signs
Weight loss, despite good appetite
Progressive weakness and muscle atrophy
Trembling
Short-based stance and short-strided gait
Excessive lying down

Diagnosis
With a horse showing weight loss, trembling, sweating and a stiff gait, despite a good appetite, this disease must be strongly considered.

Differential diagnoses
Colic – grass sickness
Laminitis
EHV-1 myelitis
Botulism

Prognosis
Very poor – most cases ultimately are euthanased. It has been reported that some appear to stabilize or improve, but none to full performance.

EHV-1 myeloencephalopathy

See Chapter 1.

Cauda equina neuritis/polyneuritis equi

A severe, chronic, granulomatous perineuritis involving the cauda equina with a milder, non-suppurative perineuritis of other spinal nerve roots and cranial nerve (especially VII and VIII) roots.

Clinical signs
Analgesia, atonia and flaccidity of:
tail
anus
perineum
rectum
bladder
pelvis

urinary and faecal incontinence
Gait defects are slight but frequently present
Cerebrospinal fluid (CSF) abnormal

Diagnosis
The clinical signs are usually definitive. With this disease the CSF reflects a
severe inflammatory response.

Treatment and prognosis
There is no treatment and a hopeless prognosis.

Neonatal maladjustment syndrome (NMS) (See Chapter 5)

The neurological disturbances are assumed to be the result of pathological
changes caused by hypoxia and circulatory disturbances.

Bacterial meningitis

Generally a fatal neurological disease, it may occur at any age but is most
often diagnosed in neonatal foals. In adults, or older foals, the cause is often
unknown, with *S. equi* cited as the commonest cause.

Clinical signs
Vary with the area of the central nervous system involved. In early stages, the
    signs are often non-specific
In general, the neurological signs worsen progressively
Initial signs – depression, anorexia and weakness
Neonates lose the suck reflex and affinity for the mare
Signs progress to cranial nerve involvement, including head tilt, nystagmus,
    strabismus, blindness, drooping lips, ears and eyelids
Proprioceptive deficits appear such as ataxia and hypermetria
Signs of severe intracranial disease, including intention tremors, recum-
    bency, opisthotonus, convulsions and coma

Diagnosis
Frequently difficult. Failure of passive transfer of immunity should increase
suspicion in neonates with neurological signs. A history of exposure to
strangles should increase suspicion in older foals or adults with central
nervous system signs.

Prognosis
Early diagnosis is essential.

11 / Notifiable diseases

The following diseases affecting horses are notifiable under the Animal Health Act 1981. The official description is that the 'diseases are subject to administrative action by the Ministry'. Report suspicion of the diseases to the local Divisional Veterinary Officer.

African horse sickness
Anthrax
Contagious equine metritis
Dourine
Epizootic lymphangitis
Equine infectious anaemia
Equine viral encephalomyelitis
Glanders or farcy
Rabies
Vesicular stomatitis

Warble fly

As there is a current eradication scheme for warble fly of cattle it is advisable to inform the Divisional Veterinary Officer, MAFF, of any cases of warble fly infection in horses.

African horse sickness

A seasonal acute or subacute viral infection of equines transmitted by biting insects enzootic in areas of Africa, with outbreaks recorded in the Middle East and southern Europe. The virus is present in the blood from onset of the febrile reaction, which is characteristic of all forms of the disease, and persists for some 30 days. Although clinically affected horses are the major source of virus during an outbreak, the current view is that there must be a non-equine reservoir host, possibly dogs, which perpetuate the virus between seasons when insects are present.

The incubation period is commonly 5–7 days but can be up to three weeks in the subacute form.

Clinical signs
The three distinct clinical syndromes all show intermittent fever of 40.5–41°C (105–106°F)

Acute pulmonary form
Initial fever
Severe respiratory signs
Paroxysms of coughing
Profuse yellow serous nasal discharge with froth
Severe sweating develops
Collapse and death
Appetite remains good until horse is unable to eat due to the laboured
    breathing

Subacute, cardiac form
Oedema of the head with later spread to neck, brisket and chest
Hydropericardium, endocarditis and pulmonary oedema found on auscul-
    tation
Cyanosis of visible mucous membranes
Petechiae under the tongue
Mild colic and restlessness common

Horse sickness fever
Fever to 41.5°C (105°F) within 1–3 days returning to normal after three days
Anorexia
Slight conjunctivitis
Dyspnoea
Clinical signs may go unrecognized
    A mixed form may be seen with a mixed strain of infection.

Diagnosis

Other than in an enzootic area it is essential that an accurate diagnosis is
made as the disease may spread to and become established in areas with
suitable insect vectors. Diagnosis based on clinical signs is possible when a
clinician is familiar with the clinical signs and lesions. With a disease that
shows in various forms, including a subclinical form, laboratory diagnosis is
essential.

Aids to diagnosis

Complement fixation and serum neutralization tests should be carried out,
the latter providing strain identification.

Post-mortem findings

Pharynx, larynx, trachea are filled with yellow serous fluid and froth
Hydrothorax, pulmonary oedema and some ascites
Subpericardial and endocardial haemorrhages are frequently present

Treatment
No specific treatment
Symptomatic treatment with careful nursing may be quite successful

Prognosis
Mortality rate in enzootic areas is 90% in horses and 50% in mules (in the latter species there is a subsequent gross debility)

Pulmonary form
Death can occur in a few hours. Should any recover, severe dyspnoea is present for a considerable period (weeks)

Cardiac form
Recovery is prolonged, with a lower mortality rate than the acute form but a fatal course may be as long as two weeks. The convalescence period is very long

Control
Vaccination using a polyvalent vaccine (not all strains included)
Remove horses from areas where insect vectors are active
Insect repellants
House horses at night

Anthrax

Caused by *Bacillus anthracis*, anthrax is usually acute and rapidly fatal.

Clinical signs

Acute form
Fever up to 41.6°C (107°F)
Central nervous system (CNS) signs of excitement then depression, respiratory distress, convulsions, coma and death within 48 hours

Subacute form
Horse may develop an intermediate acute to subacute form with several signs of colic and large spleen, palpable on rectal examination
Diarrhoea ± blood from anus
Haemorrhages on visible mucous membranes
Muscle rigidity and lameness
Tense, hot, exudative swellings on neck and lower abdomen
Terminal dyspnoea, cyanosis, coma and death in up to eight days

Chronic form
Swelling of the throat – lesions confined to the tongue and throat
Blood-stained discharges from the mouth or nose
Death from suffocation

Cutaneous form
Lesions similar to malignant pustule in man following inoculation of a skin
    wound with *B. anthracis*

Diagnosis
If anthrax is suspected, do not collect blood samples for diagnostic laboratory examination. If such samples have been taken before anthrax is
suspected they must be identified to the MAFF Veterinary Officer.

With a dead animal, a blood smear is taken (wearing rubber or disposable plastic gloves) using an ear vein, air dried, heat fixed and stained
with polychromatic methylene blue stain.

Microscopic examination of the stained smear should be carried out
under high power using an oil immersion lens. *B. anthracis* is a square-ended
bacillus with a length 4–6 times its width in short chains with a capsule.

In the horse, the organism may localize in the tonsils and intestines, as in
the pig.

Post-mortem examination
Should not be carried out on a suspected case of anthrax
Findings at a post-mortem examination of a horse which died of anthrax
    include:
    changes typical of septicaemia
    enlargement of the spleen
    multiple haemorrhages in internal organs
    effusions into body cavities
    thick dark blood

Differential diagnosis
Clostridial infection
Lead poisoning
Purpura haemorrhagica
Malignant oedema
Colic
Lightning strike

Treatment
If anthrax is suspected, do not administer medication by the intravenous
    route

Benzyl penicillin – 10 mega units i.m. every eight hours is considered the
    drug of choice. This may be followed by procaine penicillin after the
    initial loading dose (8–10 mg daily)
Streptomycin, oxytetracycline and chlortetracycline are said to be effective
    The rectal temperature of any animals grazing the same field or receiving
the same foodstuff should be taken twice daily. At the first sign of illness or
rise in rectal temperature the animal should be isolated and the use of
therapeutic doses of antibiotics intramuscularly considered.

    N.B. This is a zoonosis and every care must be taken in handling clinical
cases, suspected 'sudden death' animals and any material taken for
laboratory examination.

Contagious equine metritis

A venereal infection of horses caused by the Gram –negative coccobacillus
Taylorella equigenitalis and readily transmitted by coitus. It was first reported
in England in 1977 and two strains have been identified, one sensitive to
streptomycin and the other not.

    Control is by culture of swabs before importation or before mating.
Advice is included in the *Code of Practice for Control of Equine Reproductive
Disease* available from the Horserace Betting Levy Board, 52 Grosvenor
Gardens, London SW1W OAU. This Code is updated at regular intervals.

Dourine

A venereal disease of horses and donkeys caused by *Trypanosoma equi-
perdum*, seen in Africa, Asia, South America, south-east Europe and east
Europe. Coitus is the only method of transmission of epizoological
significance. The incubation period is between two and 12 weeks.

Clinical signs
Fever
Inappetance
Swelling and oedema of the genitalia with urethral or vulval discharge
Urticarial plaques develop on the sides of the body, in particular on the
    flanks
Progressive ataxia and paralysis, following stiffness and weakness, develops
    at a variable time after genital involvement
Extreme emaciation follows the loss of body condition and muscle atrophy

Diagnosis
The syndrome is diagnostic. The urticarial plaques are not a consistent
feature but, when present, are pathognomonic.

Diagnostic aids

Blood, oedema fluid or genital washings may be examined directly for the parasite or indirectly by the use of culture. A complement fixation test is available.

Treatment

Trypanocidal drugs have been used with variable results
Treatment should be carried out in enzootic areas at time of mating

Prognosis

The mortality rate varies, but is as high as 50–75% in Europe. In areas where
    it is much less fatal, many horses have to be destroyed
Individual clinical cases may run a 12-month course
Lifelong asymptomatic carriers do occur frequently following treatment

Control

Horses should not be imported from countries where the disease is enzootic, and the complement fixation test can be used to control importation of infected animals.

Equine encephalomyelitis

This term refers to a number of infections caused by neurotrophic arboviruses, transmitted by insect vectors, seen in North America, Central and South America, Russia and Japan. There are immunologically distinct strains of virus which vary in virulence, but all produce a similar clinical picture. The group includes the Venezuelan (VEE), Eastern (EEE), Western (WEE), as well as the Japanese (JE) and Russian Spring Summer Encephalitis (RSSE).

In general, horses responding to an infectious dose:
- develop subclinical infection
- develop encephalitis and survive
- develop encephalitis and die

It is not possible to differentiate EEE, WEE, VEE, etc., clinically.

Clinical signs

Diphasic high fever – the first febrile wave may not be noticed or it is accompanied by anorexia, weight loss and depression. The second febrile wave occurs 2–3 days later with anorexia and the onset of CNS signs which range from drowsiness to violent excitability and are progressive until collapse, prostration and death occur.

VEE in particular can present as a peracute, acute or subacute form. The peracute is very similar to that described above. The acute form shows high fever, anorexia, depression, weight loss, leucopenia and diarrhoea. The subacute form has short febrile periods.

Diagnosis
This presents a problem because of the varied clinical pictures
The place and time of occurrence and the incidence of other cases in the region must be considered
Laboratory confirmation, by examination of serial serum samples and the brain at post-mortem, is necessary

Aids to diagnosis
Virus isolation from blood or tissue
Serology

Differential diagnosis
Rabies – treat any suspect animal as if it is a case of rabies
Botulism
Leptospirosis
African horse sickness

Treatment
There is no specific treatment but good supportive therapy is justified as it may enable the horse to survive the danger period
Maintain fluid and electrolyte balances
Attempt to lower the fever – non-steroidal anti-inflammatory drugs
Protect the animal from injury with ample deep bedding or keep it outside in a paddock if the weather is suitable

Prognosis
VEE – 90% with the peracute form die within five days of the onset of CNS signs. While some animals with the acute form die, most of the subacute cases survive
EEE – 90% mortality
WEE – 50% mortality with an unfavourable prognosis when prostrate and unable to rise
More effort is justified with WEE than EEE

Control
Annual vaccination is the most satisfactory way
Protect the animal from insect vectors by housing at night and the use of insect repellants
N.B. VEE is a zoonosis with deaths recorded annually in South America.
Material from VEE cases is very likely to infect any laboratory staff handling it.

Epizootic lymphangitis (pseudofarcy)

A contagious disease of the horse caused by the fungus *Histoplasma farciminosum*. It occurs in the countries bordering the Mediterranean Sea, East and West Equatorial Africa, Sudan, South Africa and parts of Asia. This disease spreads rapidly among horses despite a long incubation period of up to 2–3 months, with horses of under six years of age most susceptible.

Clinical signs
Nodules and abscesses, with creamy pus, on the skin, predominantly on the head, neck, shoulders and limbs
Lesions on mucous membranes – eyes, mouth, nostrils and genitalia
Initial lesions may alternatively ulcerate and heal before metastasis is evident
Nodules discharge thick, oily, yellow pus
General thickening of the lymphatic vessels with nodular lesions at intervals along the vessels
Regional lymph nodes can develop large abscesses which discharge for weeks following rupture

Diagnosis
From the clinical picture.

Diagnostic aids
A smear, preferably from an unopened abscess, stained with Gram's stain will show microscopically the characteristic yeast-like cells.

Differential diagnosis
Glanders – mallein test. There is no systemic reaction and rarely pulmonary involvement as in glanders
Ulcerative lymphangitis – this is a more acute disease caused by *Corynebacterium pseudotuberculosis*

Treatment
Many therapeutic agents have been tried with little success
Excision or cleaning the abscess followed by topical iodide preparations
Destruction of the severely affected and advanced cases

Prognosis
The disease is chronic, persisting for 3–12 months with severe loss of function due to loss of body condition
Mortality rate is 10–15%

Control
Avoid using paddocks which have had clinical cases for at least six months

Isolate affected animals and decide as early as possible to destroy hopeless
cases to reduce spread of infective material

Equine infectious anaemia

A chronic disease, following an initial acute attack, caused by a retrovirus
which can be demonstrated in the blood probably for the rest of the horse's
life, regardless of clinical evidence of disease. It occurs in Europe and other
continents but not commonly in the UK.

The virus is very resistant to disinfectants and heat, withstanding boiling
for 15 minutes, but not sunlight, and remaining viable for years in blood or
the frozen/freeze-dried state.

An incubation period of 2–4 weeks is usual following natural infection.

Clinical signs

Acute form
Constant fever to 40.5°C (105°F) or higher but may fluctuate rapidly
Weight loss
Anaemia

Subacute form
Fever for periods of 1–7 days with return to normal for variable periods
Anorexia
Ventral oedema
Depression (terminally)
Jaundice or myocarditis may be seen
Weight loss

Chronic form
Recurrent febrile episodes
Weight loss
Anaemia

Diagnosis
Clinical diagnosis is difficult as it requires repeated observations
Laboratory diagnosis is possible with the 'Coggins' Test'

Differential diagnosis
Babesiasis
Purpura haemorrhagica
Leptospirosis – milder disease with spontaneous recovery in a few days

Treatment

No specific treatment

Supportive therapy including blood transfusions may assist clinical recovery

Prognosis

Acute form

Mortality rate is about 50% with the animals dying in 10–30 days

Subacute form

Periods of normal temperature followed by exacerbations of the disease until
the animal dies in 2–3 months

Chronic form

Gains weight and returns to apparently normal condition between febrile
episodes. There can be exacerbation of clinical signs at any stage

Asymptomatic carriers, following recovery from clinical disease, may
carry the virus, despite apparent clinical normality, but act as sources of
infection for other horses.

Control

Avoid taking horses from enzootic to clean areas

Coggins' Test on all imports

Limit insect vectors

Avoid mechanical spread (syringes and needles)

Suspect animals should be isolated for at least 45 days and it is preferable if
they are isolated for 90 days

Glanders (farcy)

One of the oldest known diseases of horses, still present in many parts of the
world. The aetiological agent of this contagious disease is *Pseudomonas
mallei*. The disease is far more common as latent glanders than the overt
infection, which is characterized by nodules or ulcers on the respiratory tract
and skin, usually following ingestion but also possible through wounds.

Clinical signs

Acute respiratory form

Mainly seen in asses and mules

High fever

Cough and nasal discharge with ulcers on nasal mucosa

Fulminating bronchopneumonia

Nodules on lower limbs or abdomen

Chronic respiratory form
Mainly seen in horses and commonly occurs with cutaneous form
Insidious onset
Ulcers on lower turbinates and cartilaginous septum with purulent nasal
  discharge
Chronic pneumonia – miliary lung abcesses

Cutaneous form
Predilection site – medial hock but can occur on any part of the body
Swellings which ulcerate producing dark honey-coloured pus
Lymphatics may become involved with enlargement of regional lymph
  node

Diagnosis
Very difficult from the clinical signs, in all but very advanced cases of the
respiratory form, and there should always be laboratory confirmation.

Diagnostic aids
Impression smear of the pus from fresh lesions can demonstrate the Gram
  +ve, double-walled spores
Mallein test – mallein is injected (0.1 ml) intradermally into the lower eyelid,
  the test read at 48 hours, with a positive reaction comprising marked
  oedema of the lid with blepharospasm and a severe purulent conjunctivitis
Complement fixation test

Differential diagnosis
Epizootic lymphangitis – no pulmonary involvement or systemic involve-
  ment
Ulcerative lymphangitis – no lymph node or systemic involvement
Other pneumonias or severe strangles
Infected tooth, guttural pouch infections or sinusitis may have unilateral
  nasal discharge but do not show ulceration

Treatment
Sulphonamides have been shown to be effective in man and experimental
glanders in hamsters.

Prognosis
Acute respiratory form – death in a few days
Chronic respiratory form and the cutaneous form – ill for months, frequently
  showing an improvement before they make an apparent recovery to
  persist as occult carriers, make a full recovery, or die.

Control
Quarantine infected premises
Destroy clinically affected cases
All imports should be subjected to the mallein and/or complement fixation
    test
N.B. A zoonosis generally fatal for man

Rabies

A highly fatal viral infection, generally enzootic in nature, which may
occasionally reach epizootic proportions. The incubation period is commonly three weeks but may be as long as three months.

Clinical signs
Extremely variable
Increased excitability and viciousness
Inflammation around a bite wound with the horse biting and tearing at the
    site due to the severe irritation
Depression, pyrexia, anorexia
Tremors and muscle spasm
Hind limb paralysis and dysphagia in the final stages
May be thirsty
Recumbency, coma and death

Diagnosis
Provisional diagnosis from the clinical signs.

Differential diagnosis
Botulism
Lead poisoning
Viral encephalomyelitis
EHV-1
Hepatic encephalopathy
Tetanus

Aids to diagnosis
Histopathological: evidence of encephalitis and the presence of Negri bodies
    in the central nervous system
Direct fluorescent antibody tests on brain sections
Mouse-inoculation tests with suspect brain tissue

Treatment
Isolate and keep alive as long as possible and advise Divisional Veterinary
    Office, MAFF

Do not shoot, as brain will have to be removed intact, packed in wet ice and
  sent to the official laboratory for confirmation of the diagnosis

Prevention
A number of vaccines are commercially available.

Public health considerations
Virus is transmitted in saliva – wash any saliva from skin or wound immediately. Do not handle suspect animals unnecessarily and, if this cannot be
avoided, wear suitable protective clothing. In domestic livestock the virus
can be present in the saliva for up to five days prior to clinical signs
appearing.

Vesicular stomatitis

A rhabdoviral disease that causes sporadic outbreaks of disease in the United
States, Mexico and Central and South America.
  There are two distinct antigenic strains; the New Jersey and Indiana
serotypes.
  Incubation period of nine days (3–14 days).

Clinical signs
Fever with oral lesions which cause salivation and reluctance to eat
Vesicles, then large ulcers
Tongue usually severely involved

Diagnosis
Virus difficult to isolate from blood, urine, faeces and oral swabs
Complement fixation test and fluorescent antibody test available
Serum neutralizing titres rise rapidly after infection and may persist for years

Prognosis
Generally high morbidity and low mortality rate
May be secondary bacterial disease

Treatment
Soft feed or feed made into a slurry
Fresh water at all times

12/Poisonings

Chemical and plant poisonings have a sporadic incidence in the horse. Frequently when a horse dies suddenly the owner suspects a poisoning. A suspect poisoning case should be investigated as for any other disease.

History
Frequently the most important part of the investigation. While establishing the history, by careful questioning, the veterinarian should carefully inspect any area of the yard or pasture to which the horse had access.

Clinical signs
Poisons tend to affect the central nervous system (CNS), liver, blood and gastrointestinal tract most frequently, and the clinical signs reflect the system or organ affected.

Laboratory analysis
Should only be used to confirm the presence of a suspected poison.

Before the veterinarian agrees to submit a sample, careful consideration should be given to:
1   Is there a test available and is there a laboratory willing to carry it out?
2   The cost of the test(s), which may be very high.

Plant poisoning

May follow the introduction of a horse to a new pasture or with horses grazing poor pasture with little grass growth. Horses should be removed from the pasture immediately.

Diagnosis
From the circumstantial evidence of access to plants and clinical signs, following elimination of any other cause, post-mortem evidence, chemical or botanical analysis.
1   Bryonies, buttercups, acorns – produce abdominal pain and diarrhoea.
2   Hemlock, nightshades, laburnum – produce abdominal pain, diarrhoea and nervous signs.

Treatment of the above is symptomatic and includes antidiarrhoeals, analgesics, and multivitamin preparations.
3   Bracken – Entire plant is toxic, fresh or dried, with thiaminase the toxic principle. Effects are due to myelin degeneration. Poisoning occurs fol-

lowing exposure to bracken over a long period, possibly as long as 30–60 days. The signs may develop up to six weeks after the horse has been removed from the pasture and include ataxia, weakness, incoordination, staggering, recumbency, emaciation and anaemia.

Treatment: 200–1000 mg thiamine hydrochloride i.v. and i.m.

4   St John's Wort produces induced sensitization to ultraviolet radiation (photosensitization) of the areas of the skin unprotected by melanin. It must be differentiated from photosensitization due to a liver dysfunction, where there is an accumulation of photodynamic phylloerythrin in the circulation.

5   Ragwort poisoning – see Chapter 3.

6   Yew – toxic principle is the alkaloid taxine. Death may be within minutes of ingestion.

Chemical poisoning

Poisoning with chemical agents is uncommon but may occur as outbreaks following accidental contamination of foodstuffs.

Lead

Produces a peripheral neuritis in the horse (which may be less sensitive than cattle), with general weakness, pharyngeal paralysis and pneumonia. May appear blind and head press. Anaemia with basophilic stippling of erythrocytes may be a sequel.

Diagnosis: from clinical signs confirmed by blood levels or liver and kidney levels in samples collected at post-mortem examination.

Treatment: Sodium calcium edetate by slow i.v. at 3.3 g/kg body weight in a solution of sodium chloride injection BP or dextrose BP to give a 5% solution of sodium calcium edetate, e.g. 1 ml sodium calcium edetate to 4 ml sodium chloride injection BP.

   ethylenediamine tetracetic acid (EDTA) at 75 mg/kg/day in saline for four to five days.

   Supportive therapy as necessary.

Organophosphates

Farm chemicals, e.g. dips and sprays, etc. or overdosage of chemotherapeutic product, e.g. anthelmintic.

Clinical signs include hypersalivation, excess lachrymation, miosis, sweating, diarrhoea, colic with muscular fasciculations, weakness, depression and terminal convulsions.

Diagnosis: from history of exposure, colic with signs of parasympathetic stimulation.

Treatment: atropine sulphate – approximately 1 mg/kg body weight, altering the dose to achieve the desired effect.

Anticoagulants

Either from drugs used therapeutically, e.g. warfarin, or from the ingestion of anticoagulant rodenticides. The clinical signs are those of external bleeding which is prolonged without clot formation, internal bleeding with pale mucous membranes (and colic if abdominal), and swellings under the skin, especially over joints.

Treatment: with vitamin K, synthetic less effective.

Molluscicides

Accidental poisoning by the molluscicide methiocarb has been reported. Muscular tremors, sweating and dribbling were marked and persistent with heart rate of 72 per minute and respiratory rate of 30 per minute.

Treatment: the specific antidote is atropine sulphate. Despite treatment, the horse in this report died some 12 hours after ingestion of the molluscicide.

Non-steroidal anti-inflammatory drug (NSAIDs)

Hypoproteinaemia, anaemia, thrombocytopaenia, gastrointestinal haemorrhage, renal papillar necrosis, death possible.

Treatment: supportive therapy.

Foals

   N.B. Half-life of phenylbutazone in foals is much longer than in adult horses. More serious damage to the digestive system – e.g. ulcers in the glandular part of the stomach – has been described when flunixin meglumine was administered orally, compared to erosions in this region following intramuscular injection.

Ionophores

A group of antibiotics used as potent coccidiostats in feed formulations for cattle, sheep and poultry and to increase feed conversion efficiency in cattle. The horse is particularly susceptible and great care is needed to avoid the accidental feeding of rations meant for other species.

   The most widely reported toxic effects of ionophores are associated with monensin; salinomycin poisoning has also been reported. Toxicosis may be from a single ingestion of medicated feed (LD-50 for monensin reported to be 2–3 mg/kg), or repeated ingestion of sublethal doses.

   Clinical signs are of partial to complete anorexia, ataxia and intermittent profuse sweating. It may cause acute death or delayed cardiac circulatory failure as a result of specific cardiac myodegeneration (see also Chapter 9).

   Clinical pathological findings are of toxic hepatitis and tubular nephrosis and skeletal and cardiac muscle changes. Pericardial, pleural and peritoneal effusions are usually present.

   Treatment: no specific antidotes are available. Treatment is essentially supportive, such as mineral oil to prevent further absorption, large volumes of i.v. isotonic fluids to minimize kidney damage and combat dehydration and shock. Cardiac glycosides have been found to be of little use to correct cardiac disturbances. Experimentally, vitamin E and selenium, given before pigs were dosed with monensin, subsequently produced fewer clinical signs but are likely to have little effect after toxicity has begun.

Prognosis: poor with recovery protracted and possibility of persistent cardiomyopathy and cardiac arrhythmia.

Poisoning by fungi – mycotoxicosis

Mycotoxins and mycotoxicosis are terms applied to toxic metabolites of fungal growth on food and the toxic effects produced by these compounds. Moulds grow on any stored feeds, in particular feeds with a high moisture content. A common source is from foods contaminated by moulds during the pre- and post-harvest stages of food production in Britain, or imported edible groundnut which is destined for incorporation into animal feeds.

The clinical signs vary from few, if any, to digestive and neurological disorders.

The important and immediate problem is the prevention of mycotoxicosis. Feeds that are infested or suspicious should be sampled before a decision is taken whether to use them for feeding horses. If they are to be used, irrespective of the sample results, they should be diluted with undamaged feeds to at the most 10%.

The aflatoxins are the most widely studied members of the mycotoxin family. The European Community, and individual countries, have adopted regulations restricting the amount of aflatoxin permitted in animal feeds.

13 / Miscellaneous diseases

Brucellosis

Incidence decreasing along with that in the cattle population
Generalized form:
    stiffness
    depression
    weight loss
Localized form:
    in bursae, tendon sheaths, joints, etc.
    the organism has been isolated from poll evil and fistulous withers cases.

Diagnosis
Clinical signs with known contact with brucellosis
Isolation by culture from samples
Serology – Complement-fixation test (CFT) and Coombs' test but with
    rising titre particularly significant with an SAT of 1/120, CFT of 1/20,
    Coombs' of 1/640 and above all considered positive

Treatment
Trimethoprim/sulphonamide for a month has been suggested but give
    guarded prognosis
Notify the DVO

Clostridial disease

Botulism

This is produced by toxins of *Clostridium botulinum* (often *B* but *A* to *G*
found), an organism invariably present in the soil and a common con-
taminant of animal foodstuffs. Effect follows toxins binding to neuromuscular junctions, blocking adrenal cortical hormone (ACH) release. There
had been relatively few reports of botulism in horses in the United Kingdom
until recently when there have been outbreaks involving horses fed plastic-
wrapped big bale silage and a number of single and multiple deaths affecting
horses, ponies and donkeys, all showing similar signs.

Clinical signs
The clinical signs appear 3–7 days after ingestion of the toxin and depend on
    the dose ingested

General weakness
Decreased tail/eyelid/tongue tone
Difficulty in prehension, mastication and swallowing
Development of locomotive, tongue and swallowing paralysis
Apparent ataxia
Death from respiratory paralysis

In particular the horse is seen to move with a shuffling, stilted gait, dragging its toes along the ground, and may stand with the head and neck below the horizontal position.

Diagnosis

It may be possible with some suspected cases to demonstrate the toxin in serum or digestive tract content, and this would be diagnostic proof of botulism.

The demonstration of the *C. botulinum* organism has limited significance as the organism can be found in the intestine or feed without toxin production.

The diagnosis is more commonly made following examination of the foodstuffs.

Treatment

Supportive therapy – food, liquid paraffin and electrolytes by stomach tube have been found to play an important part in cases which recover.

The use of purgatives and central nervous system (CNS) stimulants is suggested (attempts at neuromuscular treatment with neostigmine and calcium borogluconate did not show convincingly that it was beneficial) and may be counterproductive as neostigmine uses too much acetylcholine.

The horse may have been given treatment before botulism is considered as a possible diagnosis and the drugs used may potentiate the neuro-muscular blockade, e.g. aminoglycoside antibiotics, tetracyclines and pro-caine penicillin. The use of such drugs should be avoided if botulism is suspected.

Differential diagnosis

Colic, grass sickness
Lead or mercurial poisoning
Listeriosis
Mouldy corn poisoning
Organophosphorus toxicity
Viral CNS infections

Prognosis

Hopeless other than in subacute cases where signs develop slowly. Mortality has been estimated to be from 69% to more than 90%. Recovery over 2–3 weeks if occurs

Prevention

Do not feed spoiled foods or foods that are suspected of being contaminated.

The well-made clamp silage is unlikely to allow clostridial growth if the pH is between 4.2 and 4.6 with a dry matter content of more than 25%. Big bale silage characteristically has a high dry matter content and achieves a pH of 4–6. The use of added molasses to promote acetic and lactic acid production has been suggested. Only feed bag silage if the plastic wrapping is intact, the pH is 4.0–4.5, and there is a satisfactory aroma with no evidence of moulds.

Vaccination with a type specific or combined toxoid can give good immunity after two weeks and last for 24 months. Some local reaction is encountered after vaccination in horses but is seldom serious.

Intestinal clostridiosis

See Chapter 2.

Malignant oedema

See Chapter 8.

Tetanus

Tetanus is one of the oldest recorded diseases. The causal organism, *Clostridium tetani*, is ubiquitous in the environment, where it may persist for years in the spore form. Of the domestic species, the horse is the most susceptible. Infection is through wounds, which may be too small to see, including puncture wounds, lacerations, surgical procedures and mucosal ulceration.

The organism requires anaerobic conditions to be able to multiply and elaborate the two toxins produced – incubation period usually 7–21 days but can be months:

Tetanospasmin – responsible for centrally mediated muscle spasm giving constant muscle spasm with even slight stimuli giving exaggerated responses

Tetanolysin – toxic to leucocytes

Clinical signs

Progressive muscle stiffness, reluctance to move, restricted jaw movement with an anxious, alert expression

Raised tail

Prolapse of the third eyelid, especially if a sudden movement or loud noise is made in front of the horse

Dilatation of the nares

Hyperaesthesia and sweating

In more advanced cases there is a more pronounced muscle stiffness – definite 'lockjaw' signs – with all four limbs held in rigid extension

Death from exhaustion, respiratory failure or sudden cardiac arrest, by which time the horse will be recumbent

Diagnosis

Advanced cases – from clinical signs

Early cases – difficult to make a definite diagnosis but tetanus should always be suspected

Vaccination status

Differential diagnosis

Early cases:
> exertional rhabdomyolysis
> laminitis
> hypocalcaemia in the lactating mare
> CNS disease, including liver disease

Prognosis

Poor, if not hopeless, unless it is a case where the clinical signs have developed over a number of days

Mortality may exceed 90%

Cases that are very distressed or recumbent should be considered for immediate euthanasia

Treatment

Neutralize toxin – local antitoxin around the wound, systemic antitoxin intravenously. The dose varies with the manufacturer but give 100 iu/kg intravenously on the first day and 3000 iu daily for the next three days

Intracisternal antitoxin under general anaesthesia when 20–30 ml cerebrospinal fluid (CSF) is withdrawn from the cisterna magna and replaced with the same volume of antitoxin (1000 iu/ml). The horse should be supported by slings if necessary

Tranquillization:
> acetylpromazine 0.05 mg/kg intravenously
> chlorpromazine 0.4 mg/kg intravenously, 1.0 mg/kg intramuscularly

Remove external stimuli – darkened box with no noise in the vicinity

Eliminate causative organism – parenteral antibiotics with penicillins the
    drugs of choice:
    Na or K penicillin 50 000 iu/kg divided q.i.d. intravenously
    Procaine penicillin 10 000 iu/kg divided q.i.d. intramuscularly
Supportive therapy: if still able to eat, quietly feed a soft laxative diet at
    shoulder height. In advanced cases, feeding by stomach tube may be
    necessary but is frequently impossible and hazardous to the veterinary
    surgeon and groom
Intravenous feeding is expensive and rarely justified
Catheterization of the bladder and placement in slings may be necessary
    (but euthanasia should be actively considered at this stage)

Prevention

Vaccination by a primary course of two doses of tetanus toxoid given 4–6
    weeks apart, with the first booster dose of toxoid at one year and sub-
    sequent booster doses at two year intervals
The pregnant mare, previously immunized, should receive a booster of
    tetanus toxoid one month before anticipated foaling date
Suckling foals receive sufficient colostral antibodies to give protective levels
    of antibody within 24 hours of birth. The nearer to foaling the mare
    receives the booster, the greater the foal's antibody levels
Foals of vaccinated dams should not start their vaccination course until they
    are four months of age
Foals with questionable protection, e.g. unvaccinated dam or dam lacking in
    colostrum, should be given 3000 iu tetanus antitoxin within 24 hours of
    birth and at six weeks of age. The primary vaccination course with toxoid
    should start at six weeks of age
Unvaccinated horses or horses that have not had regular vaccinations (or an
    uncertain vaccinial history) can be given simultaneous tetanus toxoid
    and antitoxin products, in separate syringes at separate injection sites. A
    minimum of 1500 iu antitoxin should be given to provide immediate
    protection (within two hours)

Equine viral arteritis

Clinical arteritis has now been recognized in Britain. Transmission is by
venereal and respiratory routes.

Clinical signs
Usually apparent within seven days of infection
Very variable, ranging from a febrile response to severe disease

Most severe form
Fever to 40.5°C (105°F) for 1–5 days

Anorexia and depression
Lachrymation and conjunctivitis
Leg and palpebral oedema
Serous nasal discharge with congestion of nasal mucosa
Abortion (up to 55% of pregnant mares) possibly without clinical signs
Respiratory distress, diarrhoea, photophobia, corneal opacity and weakness
   are seen less frequently

Less severe form
Fever
Head and leg (preputial and scrotal also seen) oedema
Swollen mandibular lymph nodes
Lachrymation
Diarrhoea on occasions
Increased respiratory rate, respiratory signs frequently absent.

Foals
Anorexia
Respiratory signs and pneumonia
Colic and diarrhoea
Death possible

Diagnosis
If several horses are affected the clinical signs are seen in some or many
horses. Laboratory diagnosis is by virus isolation or paired samples to look
for raised antibody levels.

Aids to diagnosis
Virus isolation – can prove difficult in some cases
Antigen detection:
   immunofluorescence techniques are available
   complement fixation
   serum neutralization tests – have been found to be the most sensitive at
   present
N.B. No specific lesions or inclusion bodies in foetus (differentiates from
rhinopneumonitis).

Treatment
There is no specific treatment but antibacterial drugs can be used to sup-
   press or prevent secondary infection
Supportive and symptomatic therapy
Absolute rest of 3–4 weeks after the clinical signs subside

Control

Data from experimental infections suggest that the virus can persist in the tissues and be shed, particularly in urine, for several weeks after serological response. Stallions become permanent shedders

A vaccine is now available

Strict isolation of all additions for several weeks, including control of staff movements, refuse and equipment from the isolation boxes

Imports from countries where the disease is known to occur must be kept in strict isolation for a minimum of 21 days. Blood samples should be taken on arrival and ten days later for antibodies to EVA

Follow the Code of Practice for control of EVA issued by HRBLA, 52 Grosvenor Gardens, London, SW1 0AU

Hypophagia (anorexia)

May be due to depression, dysphagia or follow alimentary tract surgery.

Treatment

Offer fresh, palatable, attractive food

Check height of manger and feed bowl

Leptospirosis

Antibodies against many leptospira serotypes are commonly found, in up to 90% of horses even with no history of reported clinical signs of illness.

Clinical signs

Acute phase

Fever to 41.1°C (106°F)

Anorexia

Mild depression

Abortion possible

Icterus present if there is a significant haemolytic anaemia

Recurrent uveitis (may appear months later)

Diagnosis

From laboratory examination of blood samples (may be a retrospective diagnosis).

Aids to diagnosis

Bacteriology – culture of the organisms from the blood (acute phase only)

Haematology – leucocytosis with a neutrophilia, haemolytic anaemia may be present

Serology – acute and convalescent phase samples should be taken if possible. Indication of previous disease frequently found on routine serology as the leptospira antigens may persist in high levels for up to two years

Treatment
Penicillin and dihydrostreptomycin are the drugs of choice.

Prognosis
Good for a full recovery.
N.B. This is a zoonosis and appropriate precautions should be taken to avoid direct or aerosol contact with infective discharges, e.g. urine.

Listeriosis

A disease that occurs sporadically caused by *Listeria monocytogenes*. The organism is widely distributed in the environment, e.g. silage, water courses, sewage, etc., and entry to the animal is most probably by ingestion. The subsequent infection is dependent on the numbers of organisms ingested, physiological state of the animal and its immunological status (e.g. combined immunodeficiency foals are more susceptible).

Clinical signs
Initial loss of appetite and weakness
Fever
Increased respiratory rate and heart rate
Difficulty in feeding develops
Encephalopathies develop
Abortion may occur
Death in 3–10 days

Diagnosis
It is unlikely that a definite diagnosis will be made from clinical signs. Confirmation follows recovery of the organisms from the brain, liver, spleen and lymph nodes at post-mortem examination.

Treatment
Prompt administration of penicillin, tetracyclines or chloramphenicol at maximum therapeutic dose levels.

Prognosis
A reasonable prognosis requires early treatment
The prognosis for a horse which is showing evidence of an encephalopathy is hopeless

Louping ill

The louping ill virus is spread by the tick *Ixodes ricinus*. The horse is thought to be a reservoir of the virus with a low susceptibility to clinical infection, although encephalitis caused by the virus has been described. A serological survey in Ireland demonstrated a serum neutralizing antibody titre in 10.6% of cases.

Clinical signs
Muscular tremors
Incoordination
Progression to recumbency
Hyperexcitability and opisthotonus have been described

Diagnosis
A provisional diagnosis can be made from the clinical signs supported by the history of possible exposure to ticks. This is confirmed by serology or identification of the virus in material from the brain and cervical spinal cord taken at post-mortem.

Aids to diagnosis
Serology – complement fixation, haemagglutination-inhibition, precipitating and neutralizing antibodies demonstrated in the serum
Virus isolation – from post-mortem material

Lyme disease

Lyme disease affects many species including horses. The causative organism is a spirochaete, *Borrelia burgdorferi*, transmitted by ticks of the genus *Ixodes*. There is some evidence for additional means of transmission such as mechanical transfer by other biting insects or contact with infective urine of rodents and small animals.

Lyme disease has been recognized in humans and animals having had known contact with tick-inhabited areas in Scotland and England, more especially Cumbria, the Pennines, around Thetford in Norfolk, Salisbury Plain, the West Country and the New Forest.

Clinical signs
Clinical signs are extremely varied, with the most common sign to arouse the greatest suspicion of Lyme disease being a crippling arthritis. Other signs include cardiac conduction abnormalities, neurological impairment, or fever, rash, wasting and general malaise.

Hair loss with hypersensitivity to the tick has also been observed. It is common to have a prolonged incubation period.

Diagnosis

Serology for circulating antibodies. Horses have been shown to have a high titre without clinical signs. It is important not to overlook the possibility of Lyme disease in horses with vague, non-specific malaise or a vague shifting lameness problem, with a history of having possible exposure to ticks.

Treatment

The causal organism is sensitive to penicillin, tetracycline and erythromycin.
    Longer or higher dose therapy may be necessary
Non-steroidal anti-inflammatories
Forced rest is essential

Mastitis

A relatively uncommon condition in the mare, seen at any stage of lactation and in the dry period. A commonly isolated organism is *Streptococcus zooepidemicus.*

Clinical signs

Hot, swollen, painful mammary gland
Oedema, to a variable degree, which may extend into the perineal fold and/ or along the abdomen
Varying degree of stiffness
Inappetance
Changes in the milk

Diagnosis

From the clinical signs
The mammary secretion should be collected in a sterile container for laboratory examination

Aids to diagnosis

Direct smear – stain with methylene blue and Gram stain (after defatting the smear) for the presence of bacteria, debris and polymorphonuclear leucocytes
Bacterial culture – identification of the organism and antibiotic sensitivity tests should be carried out

Differential diagnosis

A swollen, painful, milk-distended udder immediately after weaning

Treatment

Strip out the udder, if possible, and infuse an intramammary tube of antibiotics into the gland using aseptic technique for two or three consecutive days. If possible, the gland should be stripped out frequently during the day (the 'nastier' the secretion the more important the stripping becomes), with the antibiotic infusion carried out last thing at night.

N.B. The teat ducts are very small – do not damage them by forcing tubes with large nozzles into the canal; it is possible to find intramammary tubes produced with fine nozzles.

Parenteral antibiotic may be given to supplement the intramammary infusion. With some mares it will not be possible to insert antibiotic preparations in the udder, when parenteral administration is essential.

Steatitis

Usually in young animals and often Shetlands but may occur up to 3–4 years old.

Clinical signs

Signs vary:
- May be localized
- May involve all the fat reserves
- May lead to hyperlipaemia

Treatment

Vitamin E and selenium
Corticosteroids
Insulin

Vitamin E/selenium deficiency

The location and form of deficiency symptoms depend on dietary and management factors. Foals are most often affected.

Clinical signs

If vitamin E or selenium supplies are low, muscle lesions frequently appear

If skeletal muscles are involved, the effect is white muscle disease (nutritional muscular dystrophy) with the affected horses usually becoming weak, and possibly stiff and unable to walk or rise

If the myocardium is affected, heart failure can result

Involvement of the diaphragmatic or intercostal muscles can lead to signs of respiratory distress

Hypocalcaemia (See also Chapter 8)

A well-recognized condition of lactating mares, with clinical signs seen in heavily lactating mares on lush pastures, usually within ten days of foaling. Other predisposing factors include hard physical exercise and stress associated with prolonged transport

Horses in poor condition may also be at risk.

Clinical signs

Animal is distressed, sweating, with extremely stiff, stilted gait, with hind legs held in extension

Inspiratory and expiratory dyspnoea and cyanotic mucous membranes may be present

The bladder may be very distended

Diagnosis

Can be confirmed by measuring calcium and magnesium concentrations in the blood.

Treatment

Calcium borogluconate 20% by slow intravenous injection, if confirmed

14 / Therapy

The science of drug usage is to select an appropriate therapeutic agent to use in a particular situation – or which not to use. It is likely that therapeutic failures more frequently arise from the inability to appreciate the problems of drug delivery to the site of action than from the use of the wrong drug.

Use of drugs

Routes of administration

Intravenous

Advantages
Rapid high blood and tissue levels with increased levels in areas where low levels are usually found with other routes of administration
Useful for large volumes of drugs
Useful for drugs which would be irritating or painful if given by other routes

Disadvantages
Requires good technique
Perivascular perfusion and intravenous thrombosis possible
Acute toxic reaction more common than with other routes

Intramuscular

Advantages
Ease of administration
Allows drugs to be given to achieve a reasonable blood and tissue level maintained over a period of time
Mildly irritant preparations can be given by deep intramuscular injection

Disadvantages
Only 20 ml should be given at one site
Muscle damage and abscessation possible, as is a local reaction which leaves a permanent blemish

Subcutaneous

Advantages
Although little used in the horse, it can allow large volumes to be given

Disadvantages

Drug is slowly absorbed

May produce a marked tissue reaction, in particular with thin-skinned horses

Duration of therapy and dose

Therapeutic effectiveness depends on the drug concentration, the site to be reached and the duration of administration. This means an adequate dose, given with indicated frequency over the correct period of time, using a drug which has minimal toxicity.

Special care must be taken in administering a drug that has not been licensed for the horse as there may be unpredictable results from variations in absorption, metabolism and excretion compared with the species for which it was licensed.

The drug dose rate is usually calculated on a bodyweight basis to provide good blood and tissue levels. Apparently the same product produced by different companies may vary in its formulation and/or the base used – read the data sheet.

All drug dosages given below are for guidance only and do not replace the individual product data sheet which should be consulted, in particular for contraindications and withdrawal times. All dosages are given per kilogram bodyweight unless otherwise stated.

Antimicrobial therapy

Antimicrobial therapy should be given in support of the body's natural defences. It is essential that it is used if the immune system is impaired.

Every effort should be made to confirm the diagnosis and identify the causal organism (e.g. by swabbing, tracheal aspiration, bacterial culture with antibiotic sensitivity tests of isolated bacteria), but treatment is usually started following a provisional diagnosis.

The careful selection of the antimicrobial agent to be used will reduce the total drug usage and increase the proportion of cases treated successfully. The use of a favourite antibiotic or the use of 'shotgun' therapy must be discouraged.

Do not use antibiotics as routine antipyretics, as placebos or because of pressure from clients, unless it is highly probable that a bacterial infection exists.

Antibacterial mixtures – this implies 'broad spectrum' cover, but discourages specific diagnosis and increases the possibility of adverse effects.

The effect of two antimicrobial drugs acting simultaneously on a homogeneous population is of:

1 Indifference – the effect of the two drugs (normally two bacteriostatic drugs) is approximately the same as the sum of the effects of two individual drugs. Clinically the response is little different from the end result achieved by using one effective antibacterial drug at full therapeutic dosage.

2 Antagonism – may occur with the use of a bactericidal drug and a bacteriostatic drug. It is thought that antagonism arises from the bacteriostat inhibiting the multiplication of the bacteria whilst bacteriocides are mainly effective against multiplying organisms.

3 Synergism – the combined effect of the drugs is greater than the sum of the effects of individual drugs. The use of two bactericidal drugs may produce a synergistic effect, but it is incorrect to refer to synergistic mixtures without specifying a microbial strain as no combination invariably produces this effect.

For all drugs listed below the data sheet should be consulted for special precautions, contraindications and withdrawal periods.

Suggested dosage rates and routes of administration

Antimicrobial agents

Amoxycillin syrup	20 mg/kg, t.i.d., oral, foals only
Ampicillin (Na) (trihydrate)	 7–10 mg/kg, t.i.d., i.v. or i.m. 2–7 mg/kg i.m. daily or b.i.d.
Chloramphenicol	25–50 mg/kg, t.i.d/q.i.d., i.v., succinate preferred, rapid excretion, therapeutic levels cannot be maintained. Use with extreme caution. Prolonged courses may result in reversible aplastic anaemia in horses
Erythromycin	2–3 mg/kg, b.i.d./t.i.d., i.v. 10–15 mg/kg per os t.i.d. (With rifampicin, use 15 mg/kg per os t.i.d. for four weeks or more)
Gentamicin	3 mg/kg, b.i.d./t.i.d., i.m. or slow i.v. only where tests indicate no other antibiotic effective. Foals may show severe nephrotoxicity if under four months of age
Kanamycin	5–10 mg/kg, b.i.d./t.i.d., i.m.

Metronidazole
   (Torgyl)   20 mg/kg i.v. b.i.d./t.i.d.
   (Torgyl Forte)   20 mg/kg i.m. only.

Neomycin   5–10 mg/kg, b.i.d., i.v. or i.m.,
R. equi and other susceptible Gram –ve organisms
Can be given per os to foals

Oxytetracycline   3–5 mg/kg, b.i.d., i.v., i.m.

Penicillins:
   benzyl (Na/K)   10–20 mg/kg, t.i.d./q.i.d., i.v.
   procaine   10–25 mg/kg, b.i.d., i.m.
   benzathine   15–30 mg/kg daily, i.m.
                       sub-therapeutic dose only achieved

Rifampicin   10 mg/kg per os b.i.d.
                       20 mg/kg i.v. over 3–4 hours

Streptomycin   10 mg/kg, b.i.d./t.i.d., i.m.,
only a few Gram –negative organisms susceptible

Sulphadimidine   60–150 mg/kg, daily, i.v., i.m., oral

Trimethoprim and
sulphadiazine combination:
   24% solution   1 ml/32 kg, b.i.d., i.v.
   48% suspension   1 ml/32 kg, daily, i.m.
   paste/powder   daily/b.i.d., oral

Antifungal agents
Griseofulvin   10 mg/kg, daily (i.e. 20 g of feed additive per 150 kg bodyweight)

Benzuldazic acid   0.5% solution applied topically every second day as necessary

Miconazole   0.2% emulsion (1 : 50) to lesions and immediate surrounding areas, 3–4 times daily at three–day intervals
Cream (23 mg/g) for topical use daily for up to six weeks

Natamycin   Sponge onto skin or spray. Repeat after 4–5 days. Can use to spray wood, metal, leather

Anthelmintic preparations and dosages

Benzimidazole derivatives

Fenbendazole – available as paste, liquid or granules
Routine worming   7.5 mg/kg
Trichonema sp.   30 mg/kg
Migrating strongyle larvae   60 mg/kg as one dose, or a suggested regime of
                               7.5 mg/kg daily for five days
Strongyloides westeri (foals) 50 mg/kg
Dictyocaulus arnfieldi   15 mg/kg

Mebendazole – available as paste or granules
Routine worming   5–10 mg/kg
Donkey with *D. arnfieldi*   15–20 mg/kg for five days
                               (not within four months of service)

Oxfenbendazole – available as paste or horse pellets
Routine worming   10 mg/kg

Thiabendazole – available as paste, powder or cattle pellets
Routine worming   44 mg/kg
Foals with ascariasis   88 mg/kg

Non-benzimidazole derivatives

Febantel – available as paste
Routine worming   6 mg/kg

Febantel plus metriphonate – available as paste
Routine including bots   6 mg/kg febantel, 30 mg/kg metriphonate

Haloxon – available as paste or pellets
Routine worming   50–70 mg/kg

Ivermectin – available as paste
Routine worming   200 µg/kg

Piperazine – available as powder or paste
Parascaris equorum   200 mg/kg as citrate
                               220 mg/kg as adipate
                               Maximum 30 g for foal, 80 g for adult

Pyrantel embonate – available as paste or granules
Routine worming   19 mg/kg
For tapeworms   38 mg/kg

Other drug dosages

Atropine sulphate	30–60 μg/kg (to effect in organo-phosphate poisoning) i.v., i.m., s.c.
Bromohexine HCl	0.5 mg/kg, orally 0.2 mg/kg, i.v. or i.m.
Butorphenol tartrate	0.1 mg/kg i.v. (see below also)
Clenbuterol HCl	1.25 ml of injection/50 kg, i.v., b.i.d. 10 g granules/200 kg, b.i.d., orally

Corticosteroids:
  betamethasone
  dexamethasone
  methylprednisolone
	
	1–2 ml/50 kg, i.v., i.m., 2.5–5.0 ml, i/artic.
	1–1.5 ml/50 kg, i.v., i.m. 1.0–5.0 ml, i/artic.
	20 mg/50 kg, i.m., 2.5 ml, i/artic.

Digoxin
  loading dose
  maintenance
	
	14 μg/kg, i.v., or 70 μg/kg, orally, daily
	3.5 μg/kg or 35 μg/kg

Flunixin	1.1 mg/kg, i.v., i.m., oral, daily
Frusemide	0.5–1.0 mg/kg, i.v., i.m., daily, b.i.d./t.i.d.
Hydrochlorothiazide	250 mg for an adult, i.v., i.m.
Hyoscine n-butylbromide and dipyrone	20 ml/450 kg, i.v. (i.m. can be used but local reaction possible)
Isoxsuprine	0.3 mg/kg, orally, b.i.d.
Meclofenamic acid	2.2 mg/kg, orally, daily for 5–7 days
Methadone	30–40 mg i.v. /500 kg
Millophylline	1400 g for an adult, i.m., s.c. (repeat after 8 hours if necessary)
Oxytocin	10–40 units deep, i.m.
Pethidine	up to 1 g/500 kg (see below also) i.m. best or slow i.v.

Phenylbutazone:
  horses
 	
  ponies
	
	2 g/450 kg, b.i.d., orally on day one
	1 g/450 kg, b.i.d., orally on days 2–5
	1 g/450 kg daily/on alternate days
	1 g/225 kg, daily, orally for four days
	1 g/225 kg on alternate days

Pituitary injection
  (posterior lobe)   30–100 units, i.m., s.c.

Quinidine sulphate   Test dose 5 g by stomach tube, then, if safe,
                                  give – adult 10g orally every 2 hours until
                                  cardioversion achieved (maximum total dose –
                                  80g)
                                  N.B. Wear gloves – absorbed through skin and
                                  toxic to humans

Vitamin E/selenium injection:
  adults   0.5 mg sodium selenite and 150 iu α toco-
                                  pheryl per kilogram bodyweight i.m., s.c.
                                  Repeat this dose weekly for therapy and
                                  monthly for prophylaxis
  foals   1–2.5 mg sodium selenite and 300–750 iu α
                                  tocopheryl i.m., s.c.
N.B. Do not overdose (selenium poisoning)

Vitamin K injection   Konakion (Roche) which at this time does not
                                  have a product licence for use in the horse

Drugs and drug combinations for use in sedation or assisting in the restraint of horses

Acepromazine (ACP)   up to 0.1 mg/kg, i.m.
                                  up to 0.05 mg/kg, i.v.

Chloral hydrate   3–5 g/50 kg as 10% solution i.v.
                                  3–5 g/50 kg, orally, well diluted by stomach
                                  tube or in drinking water, after withholding
                                  water for 24–48 hours

Detomidine HCl   light sedation   20–40 μg/kg
                                  moderate sedation   40–80 μg/kg
                                  profound sedation   80–150 μg/kg

In many horses the effect achieved is more profound than anticipated from the chosen dose rate. Experience has shown that the above dose rates can be reduced by up to 50% and produce the desired level of sedation.

Romifidine   40–120 μg/kg
                                  40 μg/kg for top-up

Xylazine   up to 1.1 mg/kg, i.v.
                                  up to 3.0 mg/kg, i.m.

Atipamezole (α_2-adrenergic   0.15 mg/kg
receptor agonist)

Combinations – made up in one syringe
1   Acepromazine 0.05 mg/kg + pethidine 0.6 mg/kg, i.m. or i.v.
2   Acepromazine 0.05 mg/kg + pethidine 0.3 mg/kg + xylazine 0.2 mg/
kg, i.v.
3   Acepromazine 0.05 mg/kg + methadone 0.1 mg/kg, i.v.

Other combinations
1   Xylazine 1.0 mg/kg, i.v. first, allow sedation to develop, then give the
morphine at up to 0.75 mg/kg, i.v. Acepromazine is given at the same time
(0.05 mg/kg) i.m. or 30 minutes later i.v.
2   Xylazine 0.5–1.0 mg/kg, i.v. first, allow sedation to develop, then give 0.1
mg/kg methadone i.v.
3   Detomidine HCl 20–40 μg/kg first followed by a half dose (0.05 mg/kg)
of methadone i.v.

15/Procedures which may aid diagnosis

Digestive system

Glucose tolerance test

The glucose tolerance test provides an aid to the diagnosis of small intestinal dysfunction, by assessing the monosaccharide transport mechanism mucosal integrity. It is also used to assess pancreatic endocrine function.

Method

The horse should be bedded on peat or shavings and fasted overnight, with access to water until the test commences. A blood sample is taken into a tube containing potassium oxalate/sodium fluoride anticoagulant. A freshly made 20% solution of 1.0 g/kg anhydrous glucose (or its equivalent of glucose monohydrate) in warm water, is given by stomach tube. Further blood samples are collected at 30, 60, 90, 120, 180, 240, 300 and 360 minutes after administration of glucose solution, into oxalate/fluoride tubes.

The plasma glucose levels are estimated and a plot of concentration versus time made. In a 'normal' horse the plasma glucose levels should peak

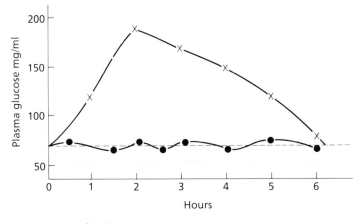

- - - - Resting level

—x— Glucose tolerance curve from mean values with a normal horse

●—● Glucose tolerance curve from mean values with a horse with malabsorption

Fig. 15.1 Mean glucose tolerance curves showing normal results and malabsorption levels.

at 120 minutes and return to the resting levels in a further 240 minutes (i.e. 6 hours from the start of the test) (see Fig. 15.1). In cases where malabsorption is present there is a flat glucose tolerance curve.

D(+)xylose absorption test

D(+)xylose is absorbed partly by passive diffusion from the small intestine and partly via the same active transport system responsible for glucose and galactose absorption, but at a much slower rate. The test can be a useful adjunct to the glucose tolerance test, particularly in cases with irregular glucose tolerance curves, despite the cost of the xylose.

Method
The horse is bedded on peat or shavings and fasted overnight. A % solution of 2.0 g/kg bodyweight of D(+)xylose in warm water is given by stomach tube. Blood samples are collected for plasma xylose estimation, using potassium oxalate/sodium fluoride as anticoagulant, before and at 30, 60, 90, 120, 180, 240, 300 and 360 minutes after the administration of the xylose.

Experimentally the maximum plasma xylose level (30 mg/100 ml) is reached at two hours, with a return to the resting level at approximately six hours. The curve obtained from the plot of plasma xylose concentration and time reflects that obtained in a glucose tolerance test with a 'normal' horse.

Lactose tolerance test

This test can aid the assessment of small intestinal mucosal damage in acute and chronic diarrhoea in foals. The continued ingestion of lactose in foals with damaged intestinal mucosa will exacerbate the clinical picture producing further fluid loss into the lumen with rapid dehydration.

Method
A 20% solution of lactose in warm water at a dose rate of 1 g/kg bodyweight is given. The procedure is the same as for the glucose tolerance test and plasma glucose levels are determined.

A typical glucose tolerance curve is obtained with the peak glucose levels of 130–170 mg/100 ml achieved at 90 minutes and a return to resting level at five hours. A flat tolerance curve indicates lactose enzyme deficiency.

Joints

Joint fluid collection

The puncture site will depend on the joint or joints affected. The site should be clipped, shaved and swabbed clean. Using strict asepsis, a short 18-gauge needle is inserted into the joint cavity (the direction of insertion should avoid damage by the needle to articular surfaces of the joint). The synovial fluid is collected with a syringe, one aliquot mixed with sequestrene for cell counts and the other collected in a clean sterile container for other investigations.

Joint irrigation

Under general anaesthesia the joint is prepared for surgery. Two 12- or 14-gauge needles are inserted into the affected joint, if possible on either side of the joint, following stab incisions of the skin with a scalpel. Sterile saline or lactated Ringer's solution, warmed to body temperature, is infused under pressure. The use of a stopcock on the underside needle is advisable to allow full distension of the joint capsule before drainage. This should be performed repeatedly to remove all the fibrin and cellular debris from the joint space and requires 5–10 litres of fluid. On completion of the lavage, the administration needle is removed, all the fluid expressed from the joint and the drainage needle removed. The skin is sutured and the joint bandaged during recovery from the anaesthesia.

Kidney

Antidiuretic hormone (ADH) deficiency

Vasopressin (available as the medical preparation only) is given in a dose of 60 units every 6 hours for a total period of 24 hours. The urine specific gravity is measured at the start and at 24 hours for evidence of urinary concentration.

Sodium sulphanilate clearance

Designed to detect renal problems in the early stages. Do not give concurrent sulphonamide therapy as it will interfere with the test.

Method
Inject 0.05 ml/kg of a 20% sodium sulphanilate solution intravenously. Collect heparinized blood samples at 30, 60 and 90 minutes post-injection for laboratory determination of sodium sulphanilate. The clearance half-time is determined from the plot of plasma concentration versus time on semi-log paper. Normal values are in the range 33–55 minutes with a mean of 39 minutes.

Water deprivation test

Used to assess the animal's ability to concentrate its urine.

Method
The horse is stabled and all sources of water withdrawn. A urine sample is collected at the start and at intervals (approximately 8-hourly) and the specific gravity determined. Blood samples are collected at the start and at intervals during the period of the test, to assess the presence of and level of dehydration, by determination of packed cell volume and total protein values (if suitable equipment is available to provide rapid results for the latter).

It is worth considering starting the test at 6 pm or later. This enables samples to be taken from the horse during the period when it is most likely to show severe dehydration and when the laboratory will be available to carry out rapid total protein estimations.

Renal biopsy

Methods
1   Following laparotomy incision.
2   Percutaneous – manipulate per rectum the left kidney against the left abdominal wall. Introduce the biopsy instrument through a stab incision, in a previously prepared and anaesthetized left sublumbar fossa. The biopsy instrument is directed into the kidney and the sample taken. The incision is closed with a suture.

The temperature, pulse and respiratory rate should be monitored for one week.

Liver

Bromosulphthalein (BSP) clearance test

This test is no better than enzyme tests as an indicator of liver damage. In the test the dye is taken up by the liver, conjugated with glutathione and then excreted.

Method
Inject 1 g of the dye intravenously. Heparinized blood samples are taken at least at 5 and 10 minutes after the injection, but more samples can be taken within the time limit if so desired. The amount of dye in each sample is estimated and the results plotted on semi-log paper, from which the clearance time can be calculated.

Do not take the sample from the same catheter or needle used to administer the dye as this will give erroneous results. The most satisfactory results are obtained by administering the dye using one jugular vein and taking the samples from the other jugular vein.

Liver biopsy

Histological examination of the liver is the best diagnostic procedure for liver disease in the horse and can aid in the assessment of the prognosis.

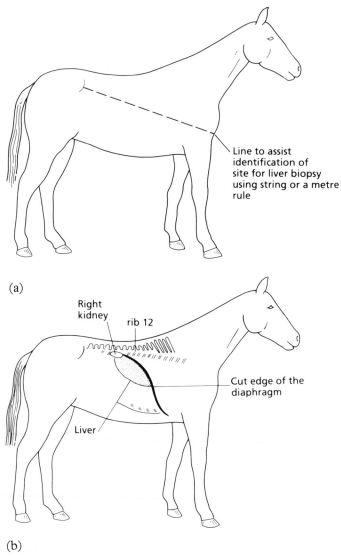

Line to assist identification of site for liver biopsy using string or a metre rule

(a)

Right kidney

rib 12

Cut edge of the diaphragm

Liver

(b)

Fig. 15.2(a) & (b) Relationship of liver as viewed from the right side to cut edge of diaphragm, right kidney and ribs.

Method

Clip, shave and swab clean an area of 5–10 cm on the right flank for

Technique 1

Local anaesthesia (5–10 ml of 2% lignocaine) is infiltrated between the 14th and 15th rib, through the intercostal muscles to the parietal pleura. Make a small stab incision in the skin, at the level of an imaginary line between the point of the hip and the point of the shoulder (see Fig. 15.2a). Pass the biopsy instrument through the skin incision, intercostal musculature (it helps to rotate the cannula at this stage) and the pleura. Ensure the stylet is in place to avoid producing a pneumothorax. Further penetration takes the cannula through the diaphragm, at which time there will be regular movement of the cannula from the respiratory movement of the diaphragm, and the liver will be encountered.

Withdraw the stylet (or trochar) and collect the biopsy sample, using a 20 ml syringe to produce a negative pressure, after rotating the cannula through 180° to the right and to the left when the cannula is approximately 6 cm into the liver. Withdraw the cannula, with the negative pressure still applied, and close the skin incision surgically and place the biopsy specimen in appropriate preservative (usually 10% formal saline) and submit for histological examination. Ensure tetanus vaccination status is adequate or administer tetanus antitoxin.

Technique 2

Block the intercostal nerves and the skin at between the 10th and 11th or the 11th and 12th ribs. Following a stab incision of the skin, introduce the cannula of the biopsy instrument, with the stylet in place through the intercostal musculature, lung and diaphragm proceeding as above (see Fig. 15.2b).

Suggested instrument

Tru-cut biopsy instrument.

Possible problems

Blood loss into the abdomen or thorax
Penetration of the bowel with a peritonitis – responds to antibiotic therapy
Pneumothorax – improper technique

Paracentesis – abdominal

Examination of the peritoneal fluid should be carried out in cases of colic and other acute and chronic abdominal disease.

Method

Clip and prepare for surgery an area of 10 cm² on the midline of the abdomen, midway between the xiphisternum and umbilicus. An 18- or 19-gauge 4 cm needle is passed through the skin, with the horse standing, and advanced through the abdominal musculature into the peritoneal cavity. Presence in the abdomen is indicated by the passage of fluid which should be collected in a sterile container and an EDTA (ethylenediamine tetracetic acid) tube. If blood or blood-stained fluid is collected, a sample of this fluid should be centrifuged in a micro-haematocrit tube and the value obtained compared with the horse's packed cell volume (PCV). Should the value be the same or very close to that of the PCV, venepuncture must have taken place and the procedure should be repeated to obtain a sample of peritoneal fluid. The samples should be sent for bacteriological and cytological examination, total white cell count and differential leucocyte count. Any delay in examination of the sample requires division of the sterile sample with the addition of an equal volume of 70% ethanol or carbowax to one aliquot immediately after collection if cytological examination is to be carried out.

Paracentesis – pleural

Strict asepsis should be observed as above. The puncture site, between the 6th and 8th intercostal space, is desensitized by local anaesthesia. The needle should be inserted close to the anterior edge of the rib, using a 16- or 18-gauge 4 cm needle and a sample of the fluid withdrawn by syringe. The samples are handled as above.

Skin

Skin biopsy

Samples should be taken, if possible, from one or two representative skin lesions.

Method

Clip and clean the area before infiltration of local anaesthetic around the lesion. Excise the lesion with a scalpel or with a cylindrical, hollow, metal punch and close the wound with a suture. If possible both normal and abnormal tissue should be included in the sample. When the sample is being taken, stretch the skin of the surrounding area. This will leave an elliptical area which is easily sutured. Place the sample in ten times its volume of preserving fluid (Du Bosq fluid or 10% formol saline) in a clean, watertight container.

Skin scrapings and hair samples

The skin scraping should be taken using a scalpel blade to a depth sufficient for the parasite expected (until bleeding occurs) with particular attention given to material at the edge of the lesion. Samples should be taken from active lesions and several other sites. Hair samples are best pulled out and any scabs present should be included in the sample (e.g. *Dermatophilus* infections).

Place the sample, or part of the sample, on a microscope slide, add a few drops of a 10% solution of KOH and heat gently. If necessary, tease out the sample in the KOH or macerate with the flattened end of a glass rod. Using a coverslip, microscopical examination is carried out using low and high power objectives.

Samples containing a significant amount of exudate may be left on a slide with 10% KOH, covered with an inverted petri dish wetted on its underside, for 12–24 hours or added to a test tube containing 10% KOH for the same period of time. In both cases microscopical examination is then carried out.

Toxicological investigations

The samples required depend on the type of toxin or poison suspected and whether the animal is alive or dead

Any tissue submitted should be at least 50 g in weight and submitted in a chemically clean plastic container

Any suspected source of the poison should also be submitted

Respiratory tract

Tracheal wash/aspiration

A technique by which samples can be taken from the lower trachea for bacteriological and cytological examination. A sample can also be taken with a suitable fibreoptoscope during bronchoscopy.

Method

Clip and prepare an area for surgery midway down the midline of the neck, between the sternocephalic muscles. After local anaesthesia with 2% lignocaine, an incision (1–2 cm) is made over the midline. Identify the trachea and pass a cannula or large bore needle between the tracheal rings into the lumen of the trachea. A long, sterilized, flexible pipe (a dog catheter), is passed through the needle and down the trachea to the point of bifurcation of the main bronchi. Introduce by syringe 20–50 ml sterile phosphate buffered saline through the tube and immediately aspirate, at the same time slowly withdrawing the tube. The sample should be divided into a sterile universal container and an EDTA tube and immediately sent for laboratory examination. Should there be any delay (e.g. sending the sample by post) in the sample being examined, divide the sample in the universal container into two aliquots, adding an equal volume of 70% ethanol of carbowax to one sample before despatch of all samples to the laboratory.

Following introduction of a fibreoptic endoscope to the caudal portion of the trachea, the above procedure can be followed using a catheter inserted through the biopsy channel.

Bronchiolar lavage

A useful technique when evaluating horses with chronic lung disease. No significant correlation has been found between the cytology of transtracheal aspirates and bronchiolar lavage aspirates.

Following the transtracheal aspiration procedure described above, the fibreoptic endoscope is advanced into either the left or right main bronchus. Five ml of 0.5% lidocaine is used to desensitize the carina and distal airways. Three 100 ml aliquots in phosphate-buffered saline should be infused sequentially into the distal airways and aspirated gently.

16 / Laboratory services

All 'normal' values given are only to be used as a guide. Each horse will have haematological and biochemical values lying within a narrow range, but for the species as a whole there is a distribution of values across a 'normal' range which varies with breed, age and type of horse, with some difference possible between individual laboratories. See Fig. 16.1.

Haematology

The sample should be taken from a horse at rest, with minimal excitement, into an EDTA (sequestrene) tube. The sample should be stored at 4°C and processed within 12 hours. If a longer time is to elapse a direct smear, air-dried, should be sent with the EDTA sample.

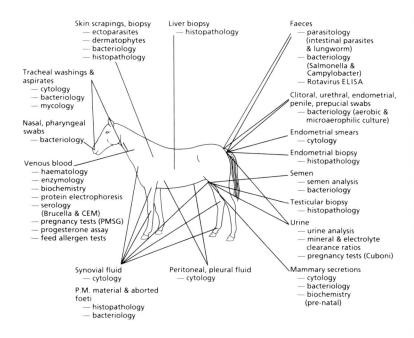

Fig. 16.1 Samples which may be taken for laboratory examination (after Beaufort Cottage Laboratory).

Reference values – a guide to 'normal' values

	Thoroughbred	*Non-thoroughbred*
Total RBC $\times 10^{12}$/l	7.0–13.0	5.5–9.5
Hb g/dl	10–18	8–14
PCV l/l	0.30–0.38	0.25–0.35

The above values can be affected by even slight excitement of the horse before or during collection of the sample. A more satisfactory assessment is made by the calculation of mean cell volume (MCV) and mean corpuscular haemoglobin content (MCHC)

	Thoroughbred	*Non-thoroughbred*
MCV fl	40–50	36–52
MCHC	34–38	34–38
Total WBC $\times 10^9$/l	6–12	6–12
Platelets $\times 10^9$/l	200–400	200–400
Neutrophils $\times 10^9$/l	2.5–7.0	
Lymphocytes $\times 10^9$/l	1.6–5.4	
Monocytes $\times 10^9$/l	0.6–0.7	
Eosinophils $\times 10^9$/l	0.1–0.5	
Basophils $\times 10^9$/l	usually absent	

Clinical chemistry

The majority of biochemical estimations are done on plasma with heparin as the anticoagulant, although serum can be used. For blood sugar estimations blood should be collected in tubes containing sodium fluoride and potassium oxalate. The samples are best refrigerated and the estimations done as soon as possible. Any delay, i.e. 24–48 hours, between sampling and estimation requires the sample to be spun and the plasma or serum removed and stored at 4°C or frozen. In the case of SDH and CK there is a significant loss in activity over the first six hours following collection and they should, if possible, be processed as soon as possible after collection.

Proteins

Total protein, albumin and globulin levels are a useful guide to general body condition, nutritional status and response to infectious or parasitic disease. The globulin fractions can be estimated by electrophoresis – α 2 (tissue damage), β 1 (*Strongylus vulgaris* larval damage), β 2 (liver pathology), γ (bacterial or viral infection).

Plasma fibrinogen

Elevated in the presence of tissue damage and may assist the diagnosis of chronic infectious or parasitic disease. Fresh, non-haemolysed EDTA and serum samples are required.

Urea

Elevated levels in the presence of abnormal renal function and uraemia. Care should be taken in interpretation of elevated blood urea levels as 'normal' horses can have levels of up to 20 mmol/1.

Creatinine

Elevated levels in the presence of renal pathology. If the urea levels are normal it should not be necessary to carry out creatinine estimation.

Cholesterol and triglycerides

Elevated levels found in the presence of abnormal lipid metabolism and hyperlipaemia.

Enzymes

Alkaline phosphatase (ALP) – Very variable levels found in the horse – unreliable on its own as a means of diagnosing liver disease

Intestinal phosphatase (IAP) – Elevated in the presence of intestinal pathology

Aspartate aminotransferase (AST, AAT, SGOT) – Elevated levels found in acute liver or muscle damage with levels peaking in 24–48 hours and returning to normal in 10–21 days

Creatinine kinase (CK, CPK) – Elevated levels found in acute muscle damage with levels peaking at 6–12 hours and returning to normal in 3–4 days

Glutathione peroxidase (GSH Px) – An indirect measurement of enzymically incorporated selenium

Lactate dehydrogenase (LDH, LD) – Elevated levels found in the presence of acute liver or muscle damage with the isoenzyme determinations required for the differentiation of skeletal or cardiac muscle, liver or brain pathology

Gamma glutamyltransferase (GGT) – Elevated levels found in the presence of chronic cirrhosis or past liver damage

Sorbitol dehydrogenase (SDH) – Elevated levels found in acute liver damage with acute extensive cell damage. Circulating levels decline rapidly after the acute damage phase is past – half-life *in vitro* and *in vivo* very short (< 2 hours)

Reference values

N.B. The clinical findings are relevant to interpretation of each test and a further sample may have to be taken and submitted for the same or for additional test(s) before a decision on the diagnosis is made. The following values are given as the values used for the interpretation of tests at the Royal Veterinary College:

Bilirubin
    total   10–50 μmol/l

Bilirubin	
total	10–50 μmol/l
	(up to 150 if stored > 12 hrs)
direct	4–15 μmol/l
BSP clearance	138–198 seconds for half clearance
Calcium	
total	2.5–3.5 mmol/l
ionized	1.5–1.8 mmol/l
Cholesterol	1–3 mmol/l
Copper	8–18.0 μmol/l
Creatinine	100–180 μmol/l
Glucose	3–6 mmol/l
Magnesium	0.6–0.9 mmol/l
Plasma fibrinogen	< 4 (adult)
	< 5 (3 weeks to adult)
Total protein	65–75 g/l
Albumin	24–36 g/l
α-globulin	8–13 g/l α_1 2–4, α_2 6–13
β-globulin	8–15 g/l β_1 8–15, β_2 6–10
γ-globulin	7–14 g/l
Triglycerides	0.12–0.35 mmol/l
Urea	3.5–8.0 mmol/l
Non-thoroughbreds	> 12 mmol/l
AST U/l	< 250
CK U/l	< 50–150
SDH U/l	> 5
GGT U/l	< 40
ALP U/l	< 250 (higher in young)
IAP U/l	< 30
GSH-Px U/ml red cells	5–30

Peritoneal and pleural fluid
Clear/pale yellow colour
Non-clotting
Leucocyte count < 10^9/l
Red cell count negligible
Protein < 20 g/l
    (Estimation of total protein can provide a quick indication of possible infection, if raised levels present.)

Bacteriology

Samples taken for clinical bacteriology should be:
1 Taken relevant to the disease (or suspected disease) being investigated.
2 The specimen must not become contaminated at time of, or after, collection.
3 Swabs taken from any site should be taken into transport medium (Stuarts or Amies charcoal) before transport to the laboratory.
4 Any specimen must be handled carefully to ensure the organisms present at time of sampling are present in the same numbers and proportions when they reach the laboratory.
5 Antibiotic sensitivity tests should be performed on any potential pathogen isolated.

Any sample of tissue or faeces should be collected in a sterile leak-proof container.

Urine examination

Urine samples should be collected into clean, leak-proof containers. If bacteriological examination is required the collection should be done as aseptically as possible with the sample collected in a sterile container.

Urine examination should be performed together with biochemical tests and both sets of results considered before a diagnosis is made. Changes may be transient and a second sample must be taken to verify any abnormalities.

Many of the tests can be carried out using dip-sticks, comparing the results with colour charts supplied.

The following should be considered:

Colour

Colour changes indicate the presence of abnormal urinary pigments and can be of diagnostic significance. The normal horse urine is more or less opaque and becomes more turbid to the end of micturition. Clear urine from a horse is probably abnormal. The reason for the abnormal colour may become evident if the sample is allowed to settle or following centrifugation, in particular if red blood cells or a white sediment indicating a crystalline deposit are found.

Odour

Requires a fresh sample for accurate interpretation. An abnormal foul odour results from excessive urine breakdown by bacteria (e.g. in cystitis).

Volume

Is of assistance in diagnosis but must not be considered in isolation. The urine volume should be measured over a period of 24 hours for accuracy. Differentiate between increased daily flow and increased frequency without increased flow.

Normal pH
Approximately 8 (7.5–9.5).

Specific gravity
1.020–1.050 (mean 1.035).

Proteinuria
Normal urine can contain very small amounts of protein, but it is at a level which is not detected by routine tests. The presence of protein (a high proportion is usually albumin) in urine indicates some pathological abnormality, but does not specifically indicate glomerular damage. The finding of formed elements, including casts, with a proteinuria increases its significance. Protein may be present in appreciable amounts in haemoglobinuria, haematuria, myoglobinuria, inflammation, toxaemia or trauma.

Deposits
Urine deposits should be examined microscopically. When normal horse urine is allowed to settle, a deposit of mucin and calcium carbonate crystals, in large amounts, will be found.

Organized deposits
Include bacteria, yeasts, protozoa, fungi, epithelial cells, leucocytes, erythrocytes and casts.

Unorganized deposits
Crystals of calcium carbonate and triple phosphate are commonly present in normal horse urine. Their presence in large numbers may suggest the possible development of urolithiasis. Urinary calculi are concretions usually formed of silicates that are contaminated with phosphates, carbonates/oxalates of calcium, ammonium and magnesium. The most commonly seen calculi are a yellow/brown colour with a rough crystalline surface composed principally of calcium carbonate. The other type found are the smooth, white phosphate calculi. Calcium carbonate crystals disappear at pH < 6.0.

Haematuria
The blood commonly causes a deep red to brown colouration to the urine but may be voided as clots. Urine containing blood will also give positive results to tests for haemoglobin, myoglobin and protein as erythrocytes are frequently lysed.

Haemoglobinuria
A deep red colouration of the urine with a positive reaction to tests for protein. Commonly it is present in the urine following intravascular haemolysis. Examine all positive samples microscopically for the presence of erythrocytes as it is important to differentiate this from haematuria.

Myoglobinuria

The dark brown colour of the urine occurs readily with the quite low levels of myoglobin in the serum. Its presence indicates a myopathy in the horse - the only notable occurrence is azoturia.

Bilirubin

When present in quantity this gives a deep green-yellow colour to urine. Bilirubin rarely appears in horse urine in any quantity even in cases of jaundice, and conjugated bilirubin is not found. Urobilinogen levels vary depending on the amount of conjugated bilirubin broken down in the intestine, e.g. extensive haemolytic damage. Bile salts may appear in the urine if flow of bile into the intestine is diminished.

Glycosuria

Most uncommon. If glycosuria is found it is essential to establish the blood glucose levels and whether glucose or reducing substances (sugars) were measured, as use of the latter may give false positive results.

Parasitology

Fresh samples in clean, leak-proof containers are required.

Despatch of samples to laboratory

Samples for despatch to a laboratory must be in appropriate containers and adequately labelled. Such containers should be leak-proof and adequately packaged to avoid damage or breakage during transport. Samples should not be despatched when they might be held up and deteriorate in the post. If the sample is urgent it should be delivered by the owner, private courier service or sent by one of the special GPO or British Rail services.

Any samples to be sent through the post must conform to the minimum packaging requirements of the Post Office. Apart from the possibility of breakage of containers in the post, spillage of contents will at the least be unpleasant and could present a public health hazard. The same consideration should be given to the laboratory staff who will have to unpack the package and, should spillage have occurred, may refuse to deal further with the specimens.

Recommended further reading

Doxey, D.L. (1983) *Veterinary Clinical Pathology* (2nd edn). Baillière, Tindall, London.
Kerr, M.G. (1988) *Veterinary Laboratory Medicine: Haematology and Clinical Chemistry.* Blackwell Scientific Publications, Oxford.

17 / Orphan foal rearing

An extremely demanding task which may be required following the death of the mare, inadequate milk production or rejection of the foal by the mare. Artificial rearing may be necessary during or following veterinary treatment.

Methods

Foster mare rearing

This can be very successful, up to 95% in experienced hands, if the dead foal's skin or amniotic fluids are available.

The mare ideally should be left in the box with the dead foal until she settles. The dead foal is then removed and replaced by the foal to be fostered, which has been starved for 1–2 hours, preferably covered with the dead foal's skin and/or foetal fluids. The mare (with her hindquarters in a corner) should be introduced to the foal and allowed to smell it before the foal is encouraged to suck by the groom. This pattern of smelling and suckling should continue until the foal is accepted, possibly for up to 12 hours. Once the mare appears to accept the foal there should still be continual observation for a futher 3–4 hours. The dead foal's skin is removed at 12–24 hours.

The finer points of introducing the orphan foal vary between yards and may include the use of odorous products on the foal and the mare's nose, restraint of the mare (manually or with sedative drugs) for some time after introduction, etc. No two introductions are the same and the success rate of some grooms appears to be much higher. The advice of such grooms, and if possible their assistance in the critical early stages, should be sought.

Bottle or bucket rearing

Mare milk substitutes include:
Specifically formulated proprietary dried milk products
Goat's milk – fed whole artificially or by allowing the foal to be suckled by a
    goat on a raised platform
Cow's milk – use low fat milk to which is added one tablespoon of white corn
    syrup and half a pint of limewater per pint of milk

The milk substitute of choice is one of the proprietary dried milk products designed for feeding to foals. Whichever product is used it should be fed little and often at a suggested daily rate of 80 ml/kg bodyweight (unless stated otherwise on the product label) with the feeding interval not exceeding 2 hours.

Supplementary feeding

A creep feed (e.g. calf quickletts or cakeletts) can be offered from ten days onwards, in small quantities replaced each day with fresh products, but consumption should be low for 4–8 weeks. Hay and clean water should always be available for older foals. Weaning can start from 15 weeks onwards.

Foals reared by hand may have subsequent behavioural problems. Exposure to other animals and groups of horses, in particular at pasture, is essential to allow development of herd instinct, ability to graze and to reduce behavioural difficulties in later life. Any behavioural and disciplinary difficulties must be punished immediately as uncorrected foals can subsequently become not only a 'handful' but also be dangerous – do not allow the foal to be a pet.

Appendix / Teeth diagrams

The teeth diagrams are a guide to the age of a horse. Other relevant factors are breed, and the time of year born in relation to the time of year at which the examination is carried out. There can be a variation of up to ± three months from the accepted 'normal eruption' or 'in wear' dates and appearance of the dental star at up to seven years of age. From seven to 14 years of age arrival of the remaining dental stars and disappearance of infundibulum can vary by up to one year.

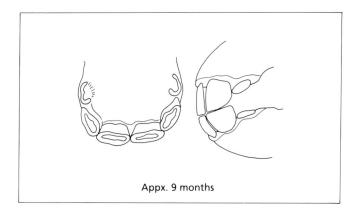

Appx. 9 months

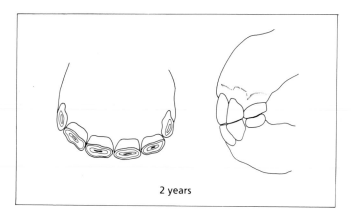

2 years

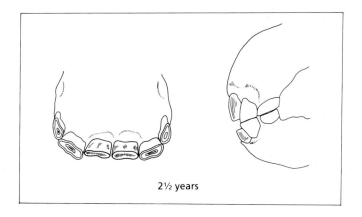

2½ years

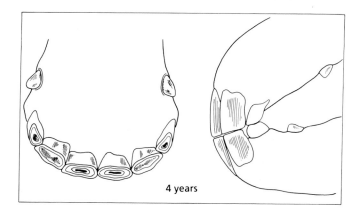

4 years

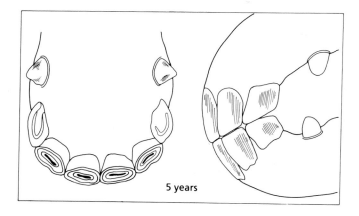

5 years

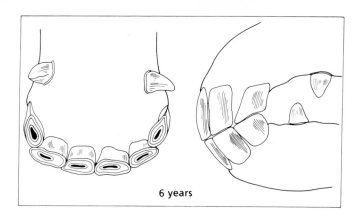

6 years

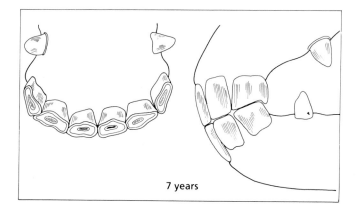

7 years

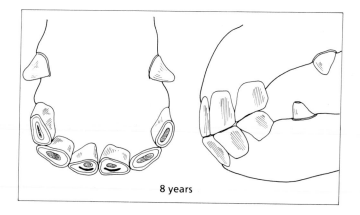

8 years

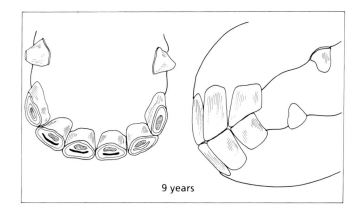

9 years

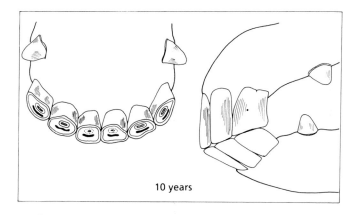

10 years

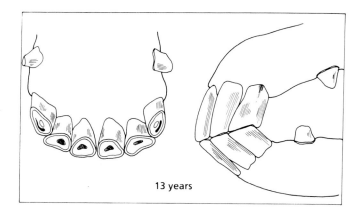

13 years

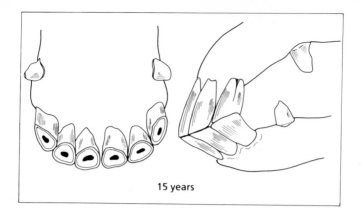

15 years

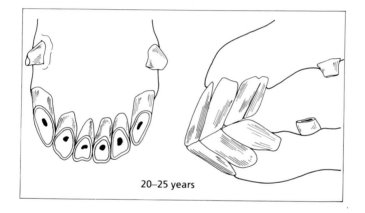

20–25 years

Further reading

Blood D.C. (1989) *Veterinary Medicine* (7th edn). Baillière, Tindall, London.
Doxey D.L. (1983) *Veterinary Clinical Pathology* (2nd edn). Baillière, Tindall, London.
Equine Veterinary Journal. R & W Publications, Newmarket.
Hickman J. (Ed.) (1985, 1986) *Equine Surgery and Medicine.* Academic Press, London.
Mansmann R.A., McAllister E.S. & Pratt P.W. (1982) *Equine Medicine and Surgery* (3rd edn). American Veterinary Publications, Santa Barbara, California.
Rossdale P.D. & Ricketts S.W. (1980) *Equine Stud Farm Medicine* (2nd edn). Baillière, Tindall, London.
Smith B.P. (1990) *Large Animal Internal Medicine.* C.V. Mosby Co., Missouri.

Index

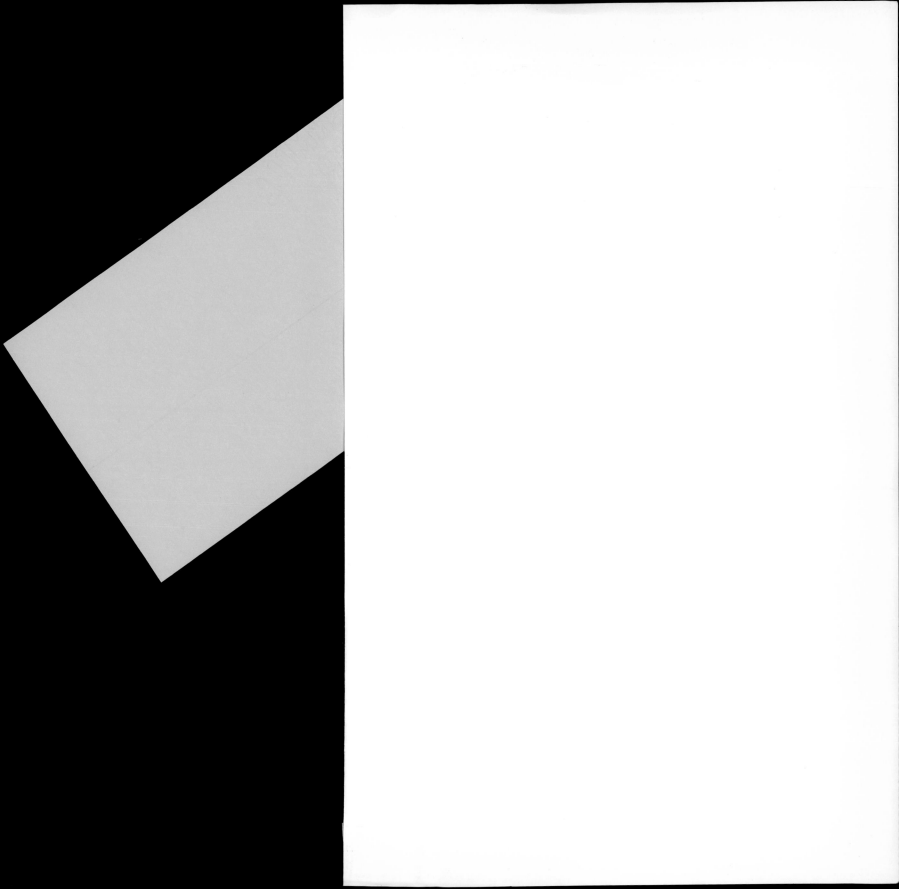